Director Liability

*A Guide to Preventing Trouble
in the Hospital Boardroom*

Robert J. Burdett, Jr.

AHA
AHA books are published by
American Hospital Publishing, Inc.,
an American Hospital Association company

The views expressed in this publication are strictly those of the author and do not necessarily represent official positions of the American Hospital Association.

Library of Congress Cataloging-in-Publication Data

Burdett, Robert J.
    Director liability : a guide to preventing trouble in the hospital boardroom / Robert J. Burdett, Jr.
       p.   cm.
    Includes bibliographical references.
    ISBN 1-55648-067-9
    1. Hospital administrators—Legal status, laws, etc.—United States. 2. Hospitals—Law and legislation—United States. 3. Liability (Law)—United States. I. Title.
KF3825.3.B87   1991
346.73031—dc20
[347.30631]   91-156
                                                                             CIP

Catalog no. 196127

©1991 by American Hospital Publishing, Inc.,
an American Hospital Association company

All rights reserved. The reproduction or use of this book in any form or in any information storage or retrieval system is forbidden without the express written permission of the publisher.

Printed in the USA

AHA is a service mark of the American Hospital Association used under license by American Hospital Publishing, Inc.

Text set in English Times
3M—04/91—0292

Richard Hill, Project Editor
Marcia Bottoms, Managing Editor
Peggy DuMais, Production Coordinator
Marcia Vecchione, Cheryl Kusek, Designers
Brian Schenk, Books Division Director

Contents

About the Author iv
List of Figures v
Acknowledgments vii
Chapter 1.   Introduction 1
Chapter 2.   An Overview of Director Liability in America 7
Chapter 3.   The Legal Basis of Hospital Director Liability 25
Chapter 4.   The "Three Eyes": Immunity, Indemnity,
             and Insurance 47
Chapter 5.   Medical Staff Credentialing 65
Chapter 6.   Corporate Asset Transactions: Mergers, Sales,
             and Asset Transfers 81
Chapter 7.   Conflicts, Compliance, and Board Risk Management ... 97
Chapter 8.   Five Commandments of Hospital Governance 109
Appendix A. Standards for Hospital Governing Bodies
             from the Joint Commission on Accreditation
             of Healthcare Organizations 119
Appendix B. State Statutes That Provide Immunity (Either
             Directly or Indirectly) for Directors or Trustees
             of Hospital Boards 125
Appendix C. State Statutes That Provide Immunity for Members
             of Peer Review Committees 131

About the Author

Robert J. Burdett, Jr., is president of R. J. Burdett & Associates, an educational and management consulting firm located in Oak Park, Illinois. He is a lifetime trustee of Bethany Hospital, Chicago, and an active trustee of Oak Park Hospital, Oak Park. He is a former general counsel of the Illinois Hospital Association and of Evangelical Health Systems, Oak Brook.

Mr. Burdett received his bachelor's degree from Indiana University in 1964 and his law degree from Northwestern University School of Law in 1969. He served as a Peace Corps volunteer in Panama from 1964 to 1966. *Director Liability: A Guide to Preventing Trouble in the Hospital Boardroom* is Mr. Burdett's first book.

List of Figures

Figure 4-1. Jurisdictions with Corporation Laws Providing Some Form of Immunity for the Directors of Private, Not-for-Profit Hospital Corporations 49

Figure 4-2. Principal Conditions to and Limitations on Immunity for Directors of Private, Not-for-Profit Hospital Corporations 50

Figure 4-3. Jurisdictions That Provide Some Level of Immunity from Liability for Members of Medical Peer Review Committees 53

Figure 5-1. Sample Questionnaire to Determine Board Views on the Importance of Various Activities 68

Figure 5-2. Sample Bar Graph Rating the Importance of Board Functions 69

Figure 5-3. Sample Bar Graph Comparing the Importance Ratings in Figure 5-2 with Time Spent on Board Functions 70

Figure 7-1. Sample Risk Management Checklist for the Board to Minimize Personal Liability Exposure 105

v

Acknowledgments

My thanks go to the many colleagues and clients with whom it has been my privilege to work over the years. With regard to the creation of this book, I particularly want to acknowledge Richard Hill, project editor at American Hospital Publishing, Inc., without whose support, encouragement, and highly professional editing this book would never have seen the light of day; Maureen Mudron and Susan Keitges, who provided superb assistance with the legal research; Larry Singer, who helped in many ways to move me toward publication; Sr. Alice Drewek and my other colleagues, past and present, on the board and management of Oak Park Hospital and at Wheaton Franciscan Services, who have provided me with countless insights into boardsmanship and hospital governance; and James Gizzi, Bradford Buxton, Mitchell Wiet, John Tighe, and Nora O'Malley, all of whom contributed their review and comments to an earlier work that provided the inspiration for this book.

I also want to acknowledge the following people for their support and positive influence on my professional and personal life: my dear father, a lawyer's lawyer who taught me to think and write; my mother, who taught me the value of love and honesty; Rev. Paul Umbeck, John King, and Stephen Kasbeer, all of whom were important mentors in my formative years; Dennis Horan, a great lawyer and moral leader who, before his untimely death, took me under his wing and opened new vistas; my children Billy, Teddy, and Caroline, who, individually and collectively, amaze me, inspire me, and give me hope for the world's future; and my wife Linda, who, since we met in 1967, has shared her life and given me more love, support, and compassion than I deserve or could ever repay.

Chapter 1

Introduction

This book is not written for legal scholars. You won't find very many cases of law and citations, so if that's what you're looking for, this book is probably not for you.

This book is written for trustees and directors of hospitals of all kinds—for-profit, not-for-profit, and public—although it doesn't get into shareholder issues that plague the directors of many business corporations. The book is short, and it is intended to give the people in charge of hospital governance a good, quick sense of what is going on in the world of hospital director liability.

For many of these people, liability is a pretty scary subject, not necessarily because of what has actually happened to them and to people they know, but because of what they have heard or seen in the general news media and of what they have read in the health care press. Director liability is also a confusing topic. It deals with areas of the law that most people don't cross in their everyday lives, and it has not been dealt with thoroughly in any other book targeted directly at hospital boards.

The task of describing difficult and confusing legal issues in an accurate and readable manner is formidable. Most books and articles that attempt to give more than superficial treatment of the subject of director liability are written by lawyers, people like the author of this book. But no matter how hard most lawyers try, we end up writing in legalese. Our oldest habits are the toughest to break.

This author has tried not to do that. The tone of this book, it is hoped, is more conversational than scholarly, more intimate than standoffish. No attempt is made to turn the reader into a lawyer. The simple hope is that the reader will learn some useful things about director liability and will come away from this book feeling better prepared and more confident about being a hospital director in a society that likes to sue.

For American hospitals, which are facing a turning point in history, this is an important goal, for now, more than ever, they need expertise and leadership in governance. There is concern in the hospital industry that fear of liability for serving in governance may cause present and future generations of directors to steer away from hospital board participation.

Whether this concern is well founded or not in the case of hospital governance is hard to determine. Most American hospitals are charitable, nonprofit organizations, and most of the members of their governing boards serve in a strictly voluntary capacity. Their only reward is the gratification they receive from service to their communities. Their motivation for this voluntary service may not invite the kind of risk-benefit analysis that can enter into a person's decision to serve for pay on the board of a business corporation.

But if the experience of business corporations in recent years serves as any guide in the hospital setting, the message is chilling. The perceived or real threat of personal liability has caused directors, especially outside directors whose skill and independence are so needed, to flee the corporate ship, as when Armada Corporation lost 8 of its 10 directors, Continental Steel lost 8 of its 12 directors, and South Texas Drilling lost 3 of its 16 directors. Similar situations occurred around the country at the height of the most recent director liability scare.

If people with skill, knowledge, and experience refuse to serve on corporate boards, the question is, who will play the director's role? The answer here may also be found on the boards of American business. Increasingly, board slots are filled by management personnel—inside directors—who frequently lack the broader view and objectivity brought by directors from the outside. Or outside director positions are increasingly filled by less-qualified and sometimes "judgment-proof" persons whose lower level of personal accomplishment may eventually be reflected in board performance.[1]

To the extent that these trends are real in American business corporations, they are not good. Have they hit the hospital sector? Perhaps not. But directors of hospital corporations have valid cause to be concerned over personal liability growing out of their board participation, valid motivation to educate themselves concerning this danger, and valid reason to do everything in their power to prevent or protect themselves against the corporate director personal liability virus that has invaded our society.

These concerns bring us to the purpose of this book. In the following chapters we look at the general liability climate as it affects the directors of American hospital corporations, examine the legal duties of hospital directors (breach of which can result in personal liability), and describe some important protections that the law provides to help shield directors against liability. We also look at what directors can do to prevent liability from ever arising, especially in the areas of hospital board involvement that most frequently produce legal claims involving directors.

The Terms Director *and* Trustee

Before tearing into these matters, however, the reader should understand a few things that are peculiar to this book. The first has to do with what is meant by *hospital director* and *hospital trustee*. In this and the following chapters, the term *hospital director* is used generically. It applies to members of the board in all corporate settings: for-profit (or business), not-for-profit, and public corporations. However, the term *hospital trustee* is used to refer only to the directors of not-for-profit and public corporations.

From the author's point of view, there is not really much reason to use the term *trustee* at all. It is done here because directors of not-for-profit and public corporations often refer to themselves as trustees and are perhaps more comfortable or pleased with the term. And for the author, being able to use different words to say the same thing helps to provide a little verbal texture. It makes writing and, it is hoped, reading a little nicer.

The Concept of Director and Officer Liability

Another thing the reader might wonder about in traveling through these pages is why there is practically no mention of officer liability, because director and officer liability are almost always mentioned in the same breath, as a single phrase. An inadequate answer to this inquiry would be that the author has chosen to write only about the liability of corporate directors. However, this rhetorical inquiry invites the author to ask, "What do you, reader, mean by 'officers'? Do you mean management officers, like your hospital's president and chief executive officer? Or do you mean board officers, like your treasurer or chairperson?"

The officers of the board are, of course, most often directors. As board officers they may have certain special duties under the law, and violation of these special duties might give rise to personal liability. But the information about director liability scattered over the following pages applies in its entirety to directors who serve as board officers. In this respect the book does deal with the subject of board officer liability. It just doesn't use the phrase *director and officer liability,* which is largely an economy of words that the author hopes the reader will appreciate. The liability of management officers—who are employees really—is a different subject, and it is not treated in this book.

Case Studies

Case studies are a great way to illustrate difficult concepts, and the reader will stumble across lots of them in this book. Except for one instance, which is clearly noted, the case studies and the names used are fictitious. There are two reasons for this approach, the first of which is very fortunate for hospital directors—there are very few real reported legal cases involving these folks or at least not enough to provide examples for the points made in this book. Thus, the author has felt a fundamental need to fabricate.

The second reason is perhaps more literary. Although truth is often stranger than fiction, many legal cases result in court opinions that are dreadfully dull and that defy enlivenment when they are retold. On the other hand, fabrication permits the freedom to invent without the danger of slander and has the added advantage of allowing for a bit of foreshadowing and continuity throughout the book.

The facts and circumstances of the fabricated cases are as realistic as the author has known how to make them. It is hoped that they will help the reader to grasp and understand difficult concepts and will enliven a subject that doesn't strike everybody as being very interesting.

The Author's Point of View

Believe it or not, authors express points of view in their works, and the author of this book will share three with the reader. The first is that the risk of liability for hospital directors, at least in the not-for-profit and public sectors, is real but manageable. Palpable threats exist in areas such as corporate negligence in medical staff credentialing and asset manipulations involving hospital corporations, parents, and affiliates; and these threats require a greater level of participation, care, and independence by directors. But in the main, the directors of not-for-profit hospitals don't get sued very often, and there are protective and preventive mechanisms and strategies that provide them with a high level of safety not enjoyed by corporate directors everywhere.

A second point of view is that there is a great deal of room for improvement in the role most hospital boards play in medical staff credentialing. Watching boards in this area of endeavor is sometimes like watching young children play organized soccer. Nobody seems to understand the rules or know what positions they are supposed to play. The team that's luckiest wins. The team that's unluckiest loses. In the case of medical staff credentialing, losing means damaging suits against the hospital and possibly against directors. Sizable improvements in board performance are needed in this area.

The author's third confessed point of view is that hospital boards do not appear to be as attentive or demanding as they might be when it comes to asserting themselves and providing for their own education and protection. Especially in the voluntary sector, directors give and give, but the need for—and appropriateness of independence of—director action and the need for their protection sometimes are paid little more than lip service.

Introduction 5

In a growing number of management-dominated, multiinstitutional organizations, there is a tendency to view independent directors — people who are close to their communities and not swept up by fad frenzies that sometimes grip professional health care managers — as impediments to the dreams and schemes of the inside "experts." As very recent judicial opinions in Pennsylvania show, this is a dangerous trend for health care in this country, and directors who fall victim to the pressure to "go along" place themselves in danger as well.[2]

In the area of liability protection, disservice to themselves can also hurt directors. The law provides a good many devices for minimizing and protecting against director liability, but corporate action to maximize this protection — action that is largely under the control of hospital directors — frequently goes ignored. In a small way, this book attempts to alert directors to the need for independence of action and describes things directors should do or demand to ensure that they are provided with the fullest range of protection from liability available under the law.

At about this point, books that deal with legal issues always carry disclaimers, and for good reason. In this vast and wonderful country, with its 50 sovereign states, diversity of law is the name of the game, despite the blundering attempts of the federal government to enforce uniformity. No person should pretend to have the knowledge or qualifications necessary to advise on every law and case relevant to a subject in every jurisdiction, and this author certainly makes no pretense in this regard.

Indeed, this short and highly generalized book is intended to provide laypeople with a notion of where danger lies and what they can do about it. When real and specific legal questions arise, however, the reader must look to licensed and qualified legal practitioners in the hospital's jurisdiction for advice and guidance.

Now that disclaimers have been dealt with, the author has one final confession to make — a confession of his respect and admiration for the thousands of men and women who give their time and talent so freely and selflessly as members of hospital boards in America. This book is written for them in the hope that it will help them keep director liability at their hospitals from causing trouble in the boardroom.

☐ *References*

1. Shaw, B. Statutory limits on director liability. *Business Horizons* 32:44–50, July–Aug. 1989.
2. The School District of the City of Erie and the City of Erie and the County of Erie v. The Hamot Medical Center of the City of Erie, Pennsylvania, and Hamot Health Systems, Inc., and Erie County Board of Assessment Appeals, No. 138-A-1989, Court of Common Pleas of Erie County, Pennsylvania, *slip op.* dated May 18, 1990. *In re:* Health East, Inc., No. 1988-1297, Court of Common Pleas of Lehigh County, Pennsylvania, Orphans' Court Division, *slip op.* dated July 12, 1990.

Chapter 2

An Overview of Director Liability in America

Let's get one thing straight at the beginning. When it comes to director liability, there is a big difference between for-profit hospitals and not-for-profit and public hospitals.

For-profit corporations have shareholders with an economic stake in the performance of the company. The shareholders look to the directors of the corporation to act in their best interests, to produce profits, and to maximize the value of their stock. When they perceive that the board has failed to do these things, the shareholders have a tendency to sue the directors, and the law generally recognizes their right to do so.

Not-for-profit and public corporations don't have shareholders. Members of not-for-profit corporations are sometimes compared to shareholders, but they have no personal stake in the performance of the organization and they are not recognized by the law as having shareholder rights. In most states members are not entitled to sue the directors.

This is not to say that directors of not-for-profit and public hospitals are free to do as they please. Like their for-profit counterparts, they are subject to well-recognized duties and standards.

The difference between the two categories of directors is in their exposure to lawsuits. The highly publicized cases resulting in major director financial liability have taken place almost exclusively in the for-profit sector. But the impact of these suits—the sporadic changes in the director liability insurance market and the "director scare"—has been universal.

One reason for this universality is the difficulty of predicting the future. As you will see, the law, which currently favors directors, may be changing, and the difference in exposure just noted could disappear with the scribble of a judicial pen. It's a good bet that if such changes occur they will take place in the context of hospital corporations—for-profit, not-for-profit, and public—because these corporations are among the largest, most active, and most visible businesses in the United States today.

Director Liability—The Good News

Throughout this country, the law of corporations provides directors with a high level of protection from personal liability. In most cases, corporate directors cannot be held liable for acts committed by their corporations and will not be held liable for their own legal and authorized actions as directors as long as such actions are carried out with prudence and loyalty to the company.

Even when directors have acted unwisely or disloyally, the law typically holds that they are liable only to the corporation itself and not directly to the shareholders, the corporate members, or the general public. Consequently, only very limited categories of potential plaintiffs are usually permitted to bring suits against directors.

Furthermore, the law now provides corporate directors with a small arsenal of weapons that can be used to limit or protect them against personal liability when the safeguards just mentioned fail. Thus, the body of corporate law is intended to ensure that directors who comply with their legal duties will not be liable for the acts they commit while serving their corporations. This, in essence, is the good news of director liability.

Director Liability—The Bad News

The bad news is that the broad protections mentioned in the preceding section do not necessarily prevent suits from being filed against directors. In fact, directors are sued with increasing frequency for the acts of their corporations as well as for their own prudent and loyal actions as directors, and the suits are often brought by individuals with no recognized right to sue.

Trial courts, which should apply the principles of director protection, are often slow to disallow claims or dismiss defendant directors in the early stages of litigation, preferring instead to allow plaintiffs with a grievance to develop their cases for fuller consideration. A judge reviewing a personal injury negligence suit naming the directors of Roaring Hell Lawnmower Company, for example, might reasonably be hesitant to dismiss the complaint against the directors after seeing an allegation that reads something like this:

> That said directors knew and were aware that after introducing the new Roaring Hell Shocker! model at least 65 users were severely maimed by flying cutter blades that became detached due to the faulty blade-

mounting assembly; yet the directors decided in their meeting of August 13 that design changes proposed by consulting engineers to correct the problem should be discarded as being too expensive, that production continue as before without any change to the aforesaid faulty blade-mounting assembly, and that a new advertising campaign extolling the safety of the Shocker! model should be undertaken.

It is sometimes said that facts make the case, and judges pay attention to plaintiffs who appear to have valid claims.

Applying the Good News/Bad News Principles

This good news/bad news scenario is illustrated by the real experience of a Mississippi public hospital board. The trustees of the Southwest Mississippi Regional Medical Center thought they were doing the right thing when they voted against renewing the medical staff membership of a staff doctor who also served on their board. What they got for their efforts, however, was a painful lawsuit naming each of them as a defendant.

Members of the medical center's medical staff served as voluntary trustees on the medical center's board of directors. This practice is recommended by the Joint Commission on Accreditation of Healthcare Organizations and is a valuable means of maintaining open channels of communication within the hospital organization.

The medical center, however, was a public hospital, and a Mississippi conflict-of-interest law prohibited individuals with an economic interest in the state's public institutions from serving on its board. There is nothing unusual or surprising about such a law. Similar laws are found in most states and are meant to protect the public from self-dealing by board members of the state's public institutions. The law would clearly prohibit an employed physician from serving on the board, but would not necessarily seem to apply to independent practitioners who merely used the hospital to treat their patients.

Unfortunately for the medical center, however, a legal opinion issued by the Mississippi Ethics Commission concluded that even independent practitioners on medical staffs of public hospitals had an economic interest in their business operations. Board service by any member of a public hospital's medical staff would thus violate the state's conflict-of-interest law.

Southwestern Mississippi Regional Medical Center had two independent practitioner members of its medical staff on its board when this opinion was published. One of them graciously resigned. The second doctor, however, refused to resign, arguing that the commission's opinion didn't have the force of law and that it didn't make any sense.

Perhaps the doctor was right. But right or wrong, the board of the medical center had a problem. It could ignore the opinion of the Ethics

Commission, or it could remove the director-physician from the board and/or the medical staff. Either course of action presented the risk of a legal challenge, but the need for action of some kind was unavoidable.

The board acted in typical board fashion. It sought legal advice, gave the matter long and careful consideration, and then followed what it thought was the most conservative and responsible approach. It decided to comply with the policy of the state agency and did so by denying the physician-board member reappointment to the medical staff. Not surprisingly, the doctor sued the medical center to seek reinstatement of his membership privileges as well as compensation for the damages he claimed to have suffered owing to the loss of his hospital practice. In his suit he named each of his fellow directors as a defendant.

As it turned out, the doctor won his suit for reinstatement. The trial court found that the medical center had failed to abide by its medical staff bylaws in denying him reappointment. It offered no opinion on the validity of the Ethics Commission's opinion that had prompted the board's action. No judgment was entered against the other directors, however, and shortly after the suit was decided the doctor's board term ended.

This conclusion, however, was an anticlimax. The real action took place between the beginning and the end. The defendant trustees, of course, each required legal representation and found themselves involved in several weeks of discovery and court hearings. The plaintiff doctor remained on the board, and board meetings, which were open to the public, turned antagonistic. Both the court hearings and the regular board meetings were front-page fodder until the entire episode ended after several months. It's true that the defendant trustees suffered no direct economic liability, but who would willingly submit to such an ordeal?

It's interesting to review this case in the context of the good news/bad news principles. Directors aren't supposed to be held liable for acts committed by their corporations or for their own good-faith actions as directors, but they were still sued in this case.

Members of the general public—and the plaintiff doctor falls into this category—aren't supposed to have the right to sue directors because of the actions of their corporations, but they do sue and often their cases are allowed to go before the courts. Thus, the good news isn't really all that good. Directors may be protected in legal theory (and in actual practice they may ultimately win most of the time), but it isn't easy and it doesn't always happen.

The Director Protection Theory

Some people may question why directors of corporations should be protected from liability at all. The answer lies in the very reason that corporations exist as a form of doing business.

If a stack of cans — say spaghetti with meatballs — fell on, buried, and bruised a customer in a grocery store that you owned, you as the owner would be personally liable for the customer's injuries. If you owned the store jointly with other people, they would be liable, too. Perhaps you would be willing to accept this risk. After all, you'd be at the store all day long, you would stock the shelves, you would know your customers, and you could keep accidents from occurring and expensive claims from being made.

Such was life in the old days, before the evolution of the corporate form of business. People who owned businesses took the profits and were responsible for the mishaps.

However, this owner responsibility approach was not very conducive to the growth of business and the attraction of capital from absentee investors. A person with money to invest but no desire to participate actively in the operation and management of a business would be foolish to take an ownership interest if it could result in personal liability. Better to loan the money, spend it, or put it safely in a bank.

Enter the corporation, that is, the fictitious person and creature of the law. The concept behind the corporation was ownership without liability. A person could invest funds in the corporation and become owner of some or all of its shares. Business would be conducted in the name of the corporation.

Profits from the business would be paid to its shareholders, but only the corporation would be liable for injuries caused to others. The risk to the owner of shares would be limited to sums invested in the corporation. Beyond these amounts the shareholder would be immune. Thus evolved shareholder immunity, sacred words in our capitalist world.

An extension of this shareholder immunity applies to directors, those persons selected by the shareholders to represent their ownership interests in the management of the corporation. Directors serve as surrogate managers for the shareholders. If the shareholders are immune from liability to third parties for the acts committed by the corporation, their surrogates should be, too, even if they are in a position to more closely direct the corporation's day-to-day activities.

Going back to our earlier example, if you were the shareholder of a supermarket chain and a display of tinned mackerel, carelessly stacked, fell on a hapless shopper, you would be more or less home free. The corporation could be sued blue, but you could not be touched.

In theory, the same is true when you sit on the board of directors of the company. You can't be sued by the crushed customer, but there is a twist. You may be sued by the corporation if your actions as a board member failed to meet a duty owed to the corporation and caused the corporation harm.

Say, for example, that the board knew or should have known that the manager of that particular store had a penchant for ordering mackerel, soup, and other canned goods to be displayed in a manner likely to pin the casual shopper or browser; that the board discussed it at board meetings and treated it as a joke: "How many customers did we nail last month?" Under our law, the corporation would be justified in seeking from the responsible directors damages for the harm and losses caused to the corporation by the directors' callous disregard for the corporation's well-being. A suit for damages could be initiated in many states by a fellow director, one, perhaps, who pointed out the folly of the situation and sought board action to correct it. Most likely, it would be brought by an officer of the corporation or a shareholder.

In any event, the suit would be in the corporation's name, with the corporation as the plaintiff. Such legal actions are known as derivative suits, and in the for-profit corporate world they are the types most frequently encountered.

But we're getting ahead of ourselves. The point of this example is that, in theory, when directors are liable at all, their liability is to the corporation and not to the general public or even to those members of the general public who ultimately are harmed by the board's failure to manage effectively. Usually, these people must look to the corporation for compensation for their injuries.

The evolutionary stories of not-for-profit and public corporations are different from those of for-profit corporations, and the differences account in part for use of the term *trustee* as a synonym for *director* in these corporate settings. But as our society has marched through the 20th century, both of these nonprofit corporate forms have come increasingly to mirror the for-profit (or "business") corporation in the manner treated under the law of the states where they originated.

Directors in both the not-for-profit and public corporate sectors are responsible to and have their duty to the corporation rather than to the general public. Typically, they can be sued by the corporation or some person with a recognized right to sue in the name of the corporation, but not by members of the public at large, not even when those people have been injured by the corporation as a result of the board's careless management.

It is sometimes said that artificial immunities create actual injustices, and there are proponents for changes in the law that would make directors more responsible to the public for corporate acts or omissions over which they have control. There are other proponents for stronger protections for directors, and, especially in the not-for-profit and public sectors, these seem to have the strongest legislative support.

While the proponents bicker, however, judges tend to lend a sympathetic ear to a broad range of persons who claim to have been injured by the actions of directors. Perhaps because of this and the highly publicized suits and recoveries against directors, legal claims naming directors have proliferated despite the fortress of legal theory that would seem to weigh against the claims.

The Risk of Being Sued as a Trustee

At this point the reader may be thinking, "This is all very interesting so far. You've told me that the law seems to protect me as a director. Then you told me that I stand the risk of getting sued as a director anyway. Well, okay, I'm accustomed to being confused by attorneys, but give me the bottom line: What are my chances of being sued, and if I'm sued what are my chances of winning?"

The answer to these reasonable questions is fairly simple: It depends. Your chances of being sued are much greater if you are a director of a for-profit hospital corporation than if you serve as a trustee for a not-for-profit or public hospital corporation. Your chances of being sued — and of winning — depend on your own conduct as a corporate director and that of your fellow board members.

Your Chances of Being Sued

It will come as no surprise that litigation involving corporate directors is a growing business. Gauging the actual extent of this business, however, is an imprecise task.

Many claims made against directors never blossom into lawsuits. They are dropped or settled privately and remain the private information of the directors, their corporations, and the director liability insurance carriers that provide director and officer liability insurance coverage for the involved parties.

When lawsuits are filed and disposed of at the trial court level they usually become public information, but most of these cases escape widespread attention. This is because most judicial settlement orders and judgments are not published in legal journals and reports. Consequently, only the more notorious cases, or cases decided in Federal District Courts, come to widespread public attention at the trial level.

It is only when trial court decisions are reviewed by appellate courts that all decisions are reported in legal publications, and only a small percentage of cases ever reach this stage of continued litigation. The cases that do, however, are important in that they provide judicial interpretation of the law of director liability and serve as a patchwork guide for acceptable director conduct.

All of the foregoing is in the nature of a disclaimer, but the following conclusions can be made on the basis of the information available: The vast majority of all claims and lawsuits against corporate directors are made against the directors of for-profit corporations. With few exceptions, the suits that result in large monetary judgments involve business corporation directors.

By contrast, there are relatively few claims and lawsuits against the directors of not-for-profit and public corporations and fewer still against such directors in hospital corporation settings.

This disparity between suits involving business corporation directors and trustees of not-for-profit and public corporations is founded on the difference noted at the beginning of this chapter: Shareholders have an economic stake in the performance of the corporation, and this economic stake presents a strong incentive to sue when corporate affairs are run contrary to the shareholders' interests. This element is simply lacking in the not-for-profit and public corporation sectors.

Shareholders fight over control of the board of directors, stock valuation in mergers and sales, disclosure of insider information, inadequate shareholder disclosure, director and officer compensation, poor corporate economic performance, and more—multimillion-dollar issues that can make or break fortunes and really get the adrenaline flowing. For some of the players, litigation can be attractively profitable in its own right, and marginally justifiable nuisance suits aimed principally at forcing a settlement benefiting the plaintiffs and their attorneys play a factor in the business corporation director liability business.

Nuisance suits also play a factor in the not-for-profit and public corporation arenas. But the types of director suits in which not-for-profit and public corporations and business corporations have the most in common involve control issues and director activities that fall clearly into the category of misconduct toward the corporation.

One legal publication that reports all appellate court cases involving directors, as well as many trial court cases, is the *Corporate Officers and Directors Liability Litigation Reporter*.[1] A three-year review of this publication revealed hundreds of lawsuits nationally against directors of for-profit corporations, but only a handful of cases involving directors of not-for-profit organizations. None of these reported cases involved hospitals. The *Hospital Litigation Reporter*,[2] a relatively new publication, has never reported a suit in which directors were named as defendants.

In *A Trustee's Guide to Hospital Law*,[3] published in 1981, Arthur Bernstein cites a number of earlier cases involving hospital trustees, including a 1973 case of significance.[4] This was a Federal District Court case in the District of Columbia in which members of the general public were allowed to bring a suit alleging trustee misconduct.

Although this case sent a tremor through the health care law bar, it does not seem to have had a lasting impact on the courts of other jurisdictions in opening the door to new groups of plaintiffs. Still, it's an important case decided by a respected federal judge, and it could serve as a foothold for community members who want to sue corporate directors for injuries caused by the corporation's conduct.

One of the more interesting compilations of statistics on suits against hospital directors was published in 1988 in *Malpractice Prevention and Liability Control for Hospitals* by James E. Orlikoff with Audrone M. Vanagunas.[5] The authors report on their observations while with the American Hospital

Association, as well as on private studies undertaken in 1985 by the Wyatt Company and in 1987 by Peat, Marwick, Mitchell and Company. The Wyatt study, based on 95 hospitals between 1975 and 1983, found that 10 of the hospitals had a total of 12 directors and officers (D&O) claims filed against them in the nine years covered by the review.

The Peat, Marwick, Mitchell and Company study, completed in 1987, covered 350 hospitals. Of those, 42 (12 percent) responded that at one time or another claims had been filed against their boards of directors.

These data provide an interesting contrast to those reported in a 1989 D&O claims survey conducted by the Wyatt Company.[6] This survey included 120 U.S. hospitals, of which 115 were not-for-profit or public corporations. It showed that in 1988 a total of 37 D&O claims were made against 16 (13 percent) of the 120 hospitals reporting.

Larger hospitals accounted for the bulk of the claims activity. Forty-one of the surveyed hospitals had 500 or more beds. Ten of these hospitals (approximately 25 percent) suffered a total of 28 D&O claims. Six of the 79 hospitals with fewer than 500 beds (7.6 percent) reported the remaining 9 claims.

Forty-six percent of all claims were covered by D&O insurance. In 24 percent of the cases the hospital did not carry D&O coverage, and in 22 percent of the cases the claims fell outside the D&O insurance protection that was carried.

Although the 1989 Wyatt survey data described here suggest growth in the number of legal claims against hospital directors, the data are by no means conclusive. One reason is that the size of the survey sample is too small and unrepresentative to be statistically reliable. More important, however, is the fact that the data fail to provide important details on the allegations involved in the claims, whether hospital directors were actually named, and the outcomes that resulted in the different categories of cases. (These deficiencies will be partially corrected in a more detailed 1990 Wyatt–American Hospital Association D&O survey of 1,000 hospitals. Unfortunately, the results of this survey were not available in time to meet this book's publication deadline.)

The Wyatt studies cited here lump together claims and cases against hospital directors and officers, volunteers, and medical staff members involved in board-delegated functions. (The acts of all of these groups are protected in one form or another under director and officer liability insurance policies.) Without a detailed breakdown, it is impossible to determine which of these groups is actually the subject of a claim. Out of 10 lawsuits, as many as 7 or 8 may name doctors involved in medical staff credentialing disputes or management officers involved in employee wrongful discharge suits, but no hospital directors. Thus, the statistics may make it appear that there is heavy action in the director liability arena when this may not be the case.

The lack of useful information in the statistical data is unfortunate because, where directors are involved, the failure to describe the kind of controversy may fuel undue fear among conscientious, hard-working, honest, and law-abiding directors who would never be guilty of the conduct that most often gets directors into trouble.

And let's face it. Not all suits against hospital trustees or directors are bad or unjustified. If a director in any kind of corporate setting uses the favored position of governance to defraud the hospital corporation or profit unfairly at the hospital's expense, the corporation should have the right to recover its damages. If there is a dispute over control of the board, legitimacy of elections, or compliance with corporate governing bylaws brought about by or involving directors, the courts may be the proper place to resolve the conflict and the directors will be party to the litigation. These are not happy dramas, but there is no surprise when directors find themselves in the middle of the stage. And most directors can avoid these controversies.

The truly vexing problems arise when directors find themselves sued by an unhappy doctor or a fired hospital employee or when the business judgment of the board is brought into question. Directors who find themselves in these types of suits are often blindsided, or end up in litigation as a result of unavoidable, no-win board decisions, as in the case of the Southwestern Mississippi Regional Medical Center trustees.

What are your chances of being sued in this type of case? On the basis of the sketchy evidence available, they seem comfortingly small if you are the trustee of a not-for-profit or public hospital and have met the duties imposed on you by the law.

Your Chances of Winning a Suit

Whereas your chances of getting sued as a director depend on many variables, your chances of winning depend on one: your performance as a board member. Irrespective of the corporate setting, the law imposes three broad legal standards of conduct on you: a duty of care in managing the business, a duty of loyalty to the corporation, and a duty of obedience to the rules of the corporation and to the law itself. These standards, and a few other important wrinkles, are described in chapter 3 of this book, but their essence is as follows.

The **duty of care** requires you to apply the same level of care in managing the affairs of the corporation as a *reasonably prudent person* would apply in managing his or her own business affairs. Generally speaking, a reasonably prudent director would not knowingly permit the supermarket corporation's manager to display cans in a dangerous manner (ultimately injuring the corporation). More to the subject of this book, a reasonably prudent director would not allow doctors to practice in a hospital without first ensuring that their medical credentials have been carefully and fairly scrutinized.

A good way to understand what is meant by a *reasonably prudent person* is to imagine yourself in the witness box of a trial court undergoing your own cross-examination in a director liability suit. The plaintiff's attorney looks at you sharply and says, for example: "Do you mean to tell the ladies and gentlemen of the jury that you sat on the board of Good Buddy Hospital, responsible for managing its affairs, and that you failed to get even one appraisal before authorizing the sale of some of its most valuable property to a real estate developer who has since made millions of dollars?" Directors learn the meaning of *reasonably prudent* very quickly in trial situations. The best advice is this: Don't wait until it actually happens to you.

The **duty of loyalty** is less complex but no less important. Being loyal to the corporation means avoiding conflicts, self-dealing, enrichment, and breaches of confidentiality at the corporation's expense. It is a duty of high integrity and trust.

The **duty of obedience** is also fairly straightforward. Directors must obey the law, as it applies both to the general public and to the corporation. Obedience to the rules of the corporation—the statutes under which it is organized and its articles of incorporation and bylaws—forms an integral part of this duty.

Complying with these three general duties won't guarantee you freedom from claims and suits arising out of your participation as a hospital director, but, short of a terrible miscarriage of justice, they will ensure that you will win any case brought against you. Sometimes directors lose in lawsuits. When they do, it is because they failed to comply fully with these standards.

Areas of Greatest Risk

By now the reader may be thinking: "Well, I could be sued, but if I keep clean and I'm prudent (whatever that means), I should be able to win any director liability suit that comes my way. Still, of the things we deal with at hospital board meetings, I'd like to know which ones pose the greatest risk of exposure."

A note to directors of for-profit hospitals is in order, however, before we go on. The discussion in this section is not going to deal with shareholder issues. For you these issues would head up any list of risk areas. But you have other areas of risk in common with directors of not-for-profit and public hospitals, so don't give up. Just understand that in your case there is more to know than is told here.

Orlikoff and Vanagunas suggest that one way to identify the areas of greatest risk to hospital directors is to review exclusions commonly found in director and officer liability insurance policies.[7] They reason that insurance companies aren't stupid. The companies have private data showing the subjects that produce lawsuits, and they protect themselves by excluding those subjects from the scope of insurance coverage.

Their book lists five areas of greatest risk, four of which are stated here:

- Medical staff appointments and reappointments, including restriction or revocation of medical staff privileges
- Discrimination in employment and employee discharge matters
- Any illegal activities of directors
- Hospital pollution, hazardous waste, and nuclear perils

Other subjects, which may not appear as insurance exclusions but which are nonetheless important areas of director liability, are:

- Violations of the duty of loyalty through self-dealing, profiteering, conflicts of interest, and breaches of confidentiality by directors
- Antitrust violations
- Transactions involving corporate assets
- Failure to comply with the corporate charter or bylaws
- Violations of state corporation law provisions

Let's look at these subjects to see why they pose the most significant liability risks for hospital directors.

Medical Staff Credentialing

Doctors sue hospitals and sometimes their boards. What could be less surprising?

It's nearly axiomatic in the law that desperate people sue. When desperation is paired with the ability to afford the enormous cost of mounting a plaintiff's lawsuit, there is a greater likelihood of litigation. So doctors, whose livelihood, practice, and pride are linked to their membership on hospital medical staffs, frequently sue when they find themselves closed out.

If boards played no role in the medical staff credentialing process, board members would be less likely to be named as defendants. After all, we have already learned that, in theory, directors are liable only to the corporation for their actions as directors. Under this theory plaintiff doctors should have no right to bring suit against directors. (Indeed, most physician credentialing suits name only the hospital corporation as defendant, and not-for-profit directors are now protected from such suits in many states.)

But hospital boards are often required to play an active role in medical staff credentialing and not just in passing on recommendations. Individual directors may also serve on hearing and review panels. Their actions in this capacity may give rise to allegations of defamation, interference with contract, or other tortious personal conduct that muddies their director immunity. In any event, they enter directly into the line of the disgruntled doctor's fire of wrath.

Thus, credentialing matters are one area where directors get sued, and every credentialing denial and corrective action proceeding involving the hospital medical staff should raise a bright red flag. The board's role in the credentialing process, and what boards can do to prevent liability in this area, are treated more fully in chapter 5.

Employee Discrimination and Discharge

The factor of desperation also arises in employment matters. Where discrimination is alleged, the government often provides the wherewithal to pay the cost of litigation. In wrongful discharge matters, plaintiffs frequently find attorneys willing to work on a contingency fee basis. Thus, this is another area in which lawsuits abound. Some of these cause trouble in the hospital boardroom.

In discrimination actions against hospitals, particularly actions involving government enforcement agencies, directors usually avoid the early fray. But find a hospital corporation that fails to comply with a regulatory or court order demanding changes in employment practices, and you will likely find the board members involved as parties. Although corporations can be hit with contempt citations for failure to comply with these orders, the contempt penalties are far more effective when they apply personally to the directors of the corporation.

Directors can also find themselves involved initially in governmentally initiated discrimination cases in which discriminatory practices appear to have resulted from deliberate actions taken by the board of directors. Private discrimination suits may also allege deliberate board action and thus involve directors as defendants.

Finally we come to the employee wrongful discharge cases. Some employees with an ax to grind will sue the corporation, every manager in the hospital directory, the board of directors, and the kitchen sink, just to help everybody feel the heat and understand how badly the aggrieved former employee feels. But in some cases board involvement in a discharge episode may be so direct as to lend credence to the threat of director liability. Charges such as defamation, wrongful interference with contract, or retaliatory discharge — all individual torts — may be so closely tied to individual director involvement as to penetrate the immunity directors usually enjoy from liability for actions of the corporation.

Illegal Activities

Illegal actions taken by a board or by individuals while acting in the capacity of director clearly fall outside the protection the board is otherwise afforded. This is a genuine area of risk, but it is not one that will concern the vast majority of directors.

Hospital Pollution, Hazardous Waste, and Nuclear Perils

The primary area of risk concerning hospital pollution, hazardous waste, and nuclear perils lies with government enforcement and penalties, rather than with private actions by the public at large. The risk of director liability, especially in nonprofit hospitals, is small and usually is tied to direct and deliberate board involvement in a violation. But where director liability is found, the damages can be enormous.

Breach of the Duty of Loyalty

When directors breach their duty of loyalty to the corporation, it is the corporation (or some person entitled to represent the interests of the corporation) that typically makes the claim. Voluntary trustees of not-for-profit and public hospital corporations have an exemplary record of scrupulous conduct and are almost always above reproach. But there are exceptions, and when directors of any type of hospital corporation use their privileged positions to realize gain or advantage at the expense of the corporation, they can and should be penalized.

Thus, suits in this arena constitute an important area of director liability exposure. In few areas are individual directors better able through their conduct to control their own level of vulnerability to this exposure.

Antitrust Violations

If a hospital corporation is charged with a violation of antitrust laws, it is probable that the individual directors will not be named or found guilty as defendants. Most federal courts take the position that directors and their corporation act as a single business unit. Because the courts reason that a single unit can't conspire with itself, this intracorporate conspiracy doctrine holds that antitrust conspiracy between the corporation and its directors is, by definition, impossible. But don't take too much comfort in this generalization.

Many antitrust plaintiffs will add the names of the corporation's directors in their suits just to stir things up a bit and get everyone's attention. More important, however, individual directors have sometimes played such a central role, and have had such a strong and independent personal interest in the act that allegedly gave rise to the antitrust suit, that they are claimed, in fact, to be individual conspirators.

In the hospital setting most of the antitrust suits naming directors are brought by doctors, and because physician board members may be considered to be competitors of the plaintiff doctor, they are most vulnerable. Medical staff credentialing denials and discharges and hospital ventures that compete with physicians' practices and other medical practices form the stage for most antitrust actions in which hospital directors may find themselves personally involved.

Corporate Asset Transactions

Corporate asset transactions constitute a tricky area in which trustees of not-for-profit and public hospitals can run into the kind of trouble frequently encountered by directors in the business corporation setting.

Suppose that over the years Good Buddy Hospital has acquired property so that it could expand from 167 to 450 beds and turn itself into Good Buddy Medical Center. However, you and your director colleagues at Good Buddy now realize that in all likelihood expansion will never take place and that the hospital probably would be better served by converting that real estate asset into cash.

At your next board meeting the administrator tells you that there is great news! A developer—someone with no connection to the hospital—has offered a contract to buy the property for $750,000. There is happiness all around.

One director asks the chief financial officer (CFO) for an opinion about the price, because "Good Buddy Hospital sits in the middle of a growing community and the price sounds kind of low to me." The CFO reports, "I talked last night to a friend who sells houses, and we agreed we ought to be able to get at least eight fifty." So the contract is authorized and quickly agreed to at $850,000, and the deal closes.

It turns out that an average of three appraisals obtained later values the land at the time of contract at $1,200,000. It also turns out that a candidate for state attorney general is making hay of the issue of hospital costs and mismanagement in the state. A savvy campaign aide who lives in town learns of the real estate transaction, knows viscerally that the developer got a bargain price, and tells the candidate.

The rest of story? Appraisals are made, the loss to the hospital is noted, the incumbent attorney general is criticized roundly for failing to police the activities of not-for-profit hospitals in the state, and the candidate wins. The first act of the new attorney general is to sue the directors of Good Buddy to recover the shortfall in the land sale price.

After a four-week trial at which each director is placed on the witness stand and grilled mercilessly for hours, the jury finds that the entire board acted so recklessly that it failed to meet its duty of care to the hospital corporation. It failed to act in a reasonably prudent manner. Judgment is entered against each director to pay the corporation the difference between the sale price of the land and its appraised value.

Valuation of assets is not the only area of potential vulnerability for boards. When directors fail through their carelessness to safeguard the assets, operations, and general integrity of the corporation, they can also be held liable for the injuries the corporation suffers.

Charter and Bylaw Noncompliance

Elections of directors and officers, amendments to articles of incorporation and bylaws, and other actions that have an impact on the control of an organization create a perfect environment for director lawsuits when these actions shortchange some group or faction holding a legally recognized interest. Such suits are initiated by corporate officers or by the state attorney general or by special courts of the state of incorporation. Some states also allow directors and other persons to bring suit.

These suits are usually based on the allegation that the rules of the organization—its charter or its bylaws—have not been followed. Sometimes these documents are imperfect or outdated. They defy comprehension or lend themselves to honest differences of interpretation. In other instances a power faction simply ignores the rules and attempts to steamroll its opposition. In any event, lawsuits in this arena are far more commonplace for not-for-profit and public corporations than those alleging breach of the duty of care.

Corporation Law Violations

Every corporation is organized under the laws of some state or jurisdiction. The laws can vary substantially from place to place, and within a jurisdiction they can be very different for the different types of corporations. Business corporation and not-for-profit corporation laws frequently are broad and general when it comes to defining what directors can and cannot do. Public hospital laws are typically more specific and restrictive.

Some jurisdictions have strict conflict-of-interest laws, especially in the context of public corporations. Many jurisdictions prohibit not-for-profit and public corporations from making loans to directors and officers of the corporation. When these laws are violated, individual directors can be held personally liable for the damages suffered by the corporation.

Managing the Risks

Although the reader may be exhausted by this list of trouble spots for directors, the list itself is by no means exhaustive. Nonetheless, the notion comes through clearly: There are plenty of things for which directors might be, and occasionally are, sued.

Perhaps the next question that might cross the reader's mind goes something like this: "It seems that several pages ago the author told me that corporate directors—what did he say?—'enjoy broad protection from liability.' That was supposed to be the good news. Then he said that directors get sued anyway. That was supposed to be the bad news. Then he pointed out that directors of not-for-profit and public corporations don't get sued very often. Most hospitals fall into these categories, so I suppose that was some more good news.

"He also said that directors who are loyal, don't break the law, and act in a reasonably prudent way will win even if they are sued. That sounds like a scouting oath, but I can live with it. Then he put me to sleep with a very long list of things that could get me in trouble. Most of them make sense, but some I never even considered. I thought I was doing a nice thing when I joined my board. God knows, I spend a lot of time at it. What in the blazes am I supposed to do to protect myself?" The answer to this question lies in performance and preparation.

It's probable that the number of lawsuits against directors, including the directors of not-for-profit and public hospitals, will increase and so will the vulnerability of all directors. These things will happen not because directors will become more evil and careless, but because the trend in America seems to point in this direction.

Americans are more and more prone to sue when they're unhappy with what they perceive to be slights and injustices, and this propensity is a powerful machine. It is fueled by a judicial system that, for better or worse, has a hard time turning a deaf ear to people with good lawyers who can make even the most ragtag tale seem attractive and meritorious.

Any hospital director who would attempt to deal with the problem of director liability by ignoring it increases the possibility of falling prey. But recognizing a problem is to have it half-licked, and there is much that directors who recognize and understand the problem can do to ensure that they are never sued or if they were that they would win with a minimum of suffering.

The starting point is to better understand the duties a person assumes in agreeing to serve on a hospital governing board. The next chapter of this book discusses in greater detail the duties and standards we have already touched on.

Another thing to do is to better understand a number of protective devices that are available to boards. In this book they are referred to as the "three eyes": immunity, indemnity, and insurance. These devices are not necessarily self-activating, and directors can maximize their protection through their own governing board actions. The "three eyes" are discussed in chapter 4.

Directors can also prevent liability from arising by recognizing and paying special attention to the areas where the greatest exposure lies. Many of these areas have already been identified in this chapter, and the most important of them receive additional treatment in chapters 5, 6, and 7.

These elements of education, protection, and prevention are the basis of managing risk in every field. If you're a hospital director, they should work for you, too.

☐ *References*

1. Andrews Publications, Edgement, PA.
2. Strafford Publications, Atlanta, GA.
3. Bernstein, A. H. *A Trustee's Guide to Hospital Law.* Chicago: Teach'em, 1981, pp. 3-31.
4. Stern v. Lucy Webb Hayes National Training School for Deaconesses and Missionaries, 367 F. Supp. 536 (D.C., 1973).
5. Orlikoff, J. E., and Vanagunas, A. M. *Malpractice Prevention and Liability Control for Hospitals.* Chicago: American Hospital Publishing, 1988, pp. 101-3.
6. *Directors and Officers Liability Survey—1989.* Chicago: The Wyatt Company, 1989.
7. Orlikoff and Vanagunas, p. 105.

Chapter 3

The Legal Basis of Hospital Director Liability

There is the story of the prominent citizen who was asked to serve on the board of a local hospital. "How much time will it take?" the citizen asked. "No more than a few hours a month," the citizen was told.

"What will I have to do?" the citizen asked. "Just attend the monthly meeting of the board and do a little committee work," the citizen was told.

"Well, I've always thought highly of the hospital," the citizen said, "and I'd like to help out. I'm awfully busy with other things, but if it won't really be that much of a burden, I'll do it."

On the evening of the first board meeting, the citizen kissed the citizen-spouse good-bye and was never seen again.

If you've ever lived through your own variation of this story firsthand, you know that hospitals are big businesses and that serving as a hospital director is a big job.

Whether it is a metropolitan medical center or a rural health care facility, the American hospital counts among the largest employers and centers of economic activity within our communities. Decisions made by hospital boards can have a profound impact, not just on health care in the community, but on the community's social and economic condition as well.

And hospitals are different. Understanding what makes them tick requires long exposure and study for community members who volunteer their time to serve in governance. The unusual relationship among the independent medical staff, the hospital, and the board has no close analogy in our society. Payment mechanisms and accounting systems are unlike those in most other industries. And government regulations unique to hospitals and health care permeate every facet of the hospital's operation.

Underpayment for health care services by Medicare, Medicaid, and private insurers and intense competition within the health care sector place the institution's survival at risk. Increased scrutiny of the quality of care rendered by the hospital increases the squeeze.

And as hospital governance has gained in complexity, the vulnerability of directors to liability has grown. All of these issues and dynamics, and many, many more, are on the table every time the board sits down for its regular deliberations. Little wonder, then, that hospital directors often struggle with their roles and agonize over their own duties and performance.

Perhaps there was a time when volunteering to serve as a trustee on the local hospital board was viewed as a feather in one's cap and a position that required limited work or responsibility beyond a little fund-raising. There may still be prestige in such service, but it requires hard work. For many people this reward may not be adequate. As Joe Lewis used to say, "Everybody wants to go to heaven, but nobody wants to die."

Corporate Control and Ownership

For those who decide to take the plunge into hospital governance the first questions typically asked are: "What are my duties?" and "What kind of liability am I exposed to?" Directors also want to know what steps can be taken to protect them against any potential liability to which they may be exposed.

Legal duty and legal liability are hand-in-glove concepts. For a hospital director, legal duty is a standard of conduct found in law or contract. Legal liability can arise when that duty has been breached.

The starting point in a review of the legal duties of hospital corporate directors is the corporation itself. All corporations are creatures of the law and are governed by the statutes of the states in which they are organized.

Under these laws, the primary difference between business corporations and nonprofit corporations lies not in the generation of profits, but in the concept of ownership. Business or for-profit corporations are owned by shareholders, who risk capital and gain financial benefit from the profits and increased value of the business. Control of the corporation rests with the owners of the stock, and the directors elected by the shareholders owe a fiduciary duty to these owners and to the corporation.

On the other hand, not-for-profit and public corporations are more in the nature of public trusts. They have no private owners, and no private person is entitled to benefit in their profits and increased value. These benefits are "owned" by the corporation and held for the benefit of the public. They must be used in the furtherance of the corporation's purposes.

The methods for controlling not-for-profit and public corporations are governed by statute and have nothing to do with ownership. Control of not-for-profit corporations may be vested in a membership group, which elects directors, or in a self-perpetuating board of directors, which provides for its own succession. Control of public corporations typically vests, directly or indirectly, in elected officials. The directors in both cases owe their fiduciary duty to the corporation alone.

The Role and the Dilemma of the Board

The differences between the types of corporations aside, modern state law generally applies much the same standards of performance to all corporate directors. In virtually every state, the law requires that the affairs of the corporation be managed by, or under the direction of, the board.

Management does not mean that boards must have a hands-on role in each and every activity of operations. Boards are allowed to delegate certain of their *functions* to committees, councils, and professional managers. But the *responsibility* and attendant liability for management may not be delegated. These remain the sole domain of the board and its directors and cannot be abdicated. As long as we've already maligned the directors of our fictitious Good Buddy Hospital, let's use them as an example.

At Good Buddy the job of reviewing the credentials of medical practitioners seeking appointment and reappointment to the hospital was long ago delegated to the medical staff. Unfortunately, the Good Buddy medical staff is a cozy little group dedicated to protecting its own turf.

A busy surgeon, one of the long-standing members of the medical staff, hires an associate, a doctor with a notably unexceptional career and little independent surgical experience, to assist in performing routine office work and postoperative hospital rounds. This doctor applies for staff privileges, including full clinical privileges in general surgery.

The medical staff recognizes that this associate could be trouble if he was allowed to practice independently, but recommends acceptance anyway upon the urging of the employing surgeon. At the end of their regular board meeting, the directors of Good Buddy take just a minute to approve the various medical staff recommendations without question or comment. After all, the board delegated these credentialing matters to the medical staff, and who is the board to question such a routine credentialing recommendation?

Five months later, the new doctor severs his association with the hiring surgeon, hangs out a shingle, and starts cutting patients in Good Buddy's operating room. But not without incident. In fact, not without lots of incidents. Within a few more months, several patients had been maimed and mutilated by this inexpert doctor. Medical staff membership is terminated and the doctor goes away, but soon big malpractice suits start to hit the hospital.

Fortunately for the directors, they probably can't be sued by the patients (or their families) they have allowed to be killed, dismembered, or handicapped for life as a result of the board's blind delegation of credentialing to the medical staff. But the hospital corporation, which the directors are supposed to manage and safeguard, suffered immeasurably as a result of the suits.

Who is at fault for this fiasco? The medical staff is certainly at fault in its failure to carry out the credentialing function delegated to it by the board. But, legally, it is the board that is responsible for this failure. Delegation in the world of corporate boards just means that somebody else gets to do the job. The delegator always has the responsibility for acting in a reasonably prudent manner to ensure the likelihood that the job will be done right.

Can the board of Good Buddy face liability for its failure to exercise its duty of care? The answer is that it probably won't, but it could. The likelihood would be greatest if it were a for-profit corporation and its economic performance were damaged by this episode. Unhappy shareholders might very well bring the board to task. The paucity of eligible plaintiffs in the not-for-profit and public hospital settings lessens the likelihood of suit, but the possibility of liability remains very real.

This concept of ultimate responsibility creates a challenging dilemma for boards. On the one hand, directors are exhorted not to meddle in management, to rise above detail, and to focus on the big picture. On the other hand, the board and the hospital corporation it is entrusted to guide stand responsible for the failures of delegation, for the collapse of detail.

The solution of this dilemma is one job the board cannot delegate. The board must develop its own understanding of those issues that are so important as to warrant considerable time, knowledge, and attention. Medical staff credentialing is one of these areas, and others will be highlighted throughout the later chapters of this book.

Common-Law Duties of Hospital Directors

Although the burden of responsibility placed on boards is great, the law recognizes that individual directors cannot be held to a superhuman standard of conduct and that directors should not be held personally liable for damages except in those instances in which recognized duties have been violated. The law holds that directors serve their corporations in a fiduciary capacity. Simply put, directors must carry out their duties in good faith, serving the best interests of the corporation. Except in limited instances, today this rule is generally the same for directors of all hospital corporations—for-profit, not-for-profit, and public.

Individual director liability *to the corporation* arises when this fiduciary responsibility has been violated. The standards of conduct for meeting this fiduciary responsibility vary in nuance from state to state and are undergoing constant evolution. Nonetheless, the three standards mentioned in chapter 2 are of such universal importance that they should be familiar to all directors: the *duty of loyalty,* the *duty of care,* and the *duty of obedience.*

The Duty of Loyalty

Directors of hospital corporations are empowered by law to manage and are entrusted by society or shareholders to do so with individual loyalty to the best interests of the organization. This duty of loyalty bars directors from using their position and authority in a self-serving manner.

Competition with the corporation, *usurping* business opportunities, and *profiting* from insider information violate this duty of loyalty, are prohibited, and can result in individual director liability to the corporation. Likewise, *conflicts* arising out of a duality of interests can also breach this duty of loyalty and must be dealt with carefully.

The duty of loyalty originated in the common law, and guidance in its interpretation has traditionally been found in judicial opinions. Many states, however, are now codifying certain aspects of the duty in order to provide greater predictability as to what form of conduct is acceptable.

This movement toward codification is especially great in the area of conflicts of interest. Indeed, in the case of public hospital corporations, directors are typically placed under tight restrictions.

Outside the public hospital arena, however, the statutes generally authorize a director (or companies in which the director has an interest) to transact business with the hospital corporation, as long as the transaction is fair to the hospital and procedural safeguards that remove the interested director from participation in related decisions are met.

The importance of the duty of loyalty has long been recognized by hospitals and their directors, especially in the not-for-profit sector. Nonetheless, opportunities for violation of the duty, both intentional and unintentional, abound. Indeed, many of the *successful* lawsuits against hospital directors result from breaches of the duty of loyalty. Knowing about and acquiescing to another director's violation of the duty of loyalty might also give rise to widespread board liability.

Prudent boards adopt clear statements of policy regarding conflicts of interest and other possible breaches of loyalty. In chapter 7, we describe how these statements are regularly distributed to all directors, officers, and others in sensitive positions and that disclosure statements are required annually. These practices alert directors to the need for care and provide a means of helping directors to avoid unintentional violations.

Although policies and procedures will not protect or save a transaction that is patently in violation of the duty of loyalty or be effective in the case of a dishonest director, they will help the vast majority of honest and conscientious directors to avoid unintended breaches and unwanted liability. Without these policies and procedures in place, directors are left to follow their own impressions of what is legally required or appropriate conduct. In this era of sensitivity and this area of liability danger, neither the corporation nor its directors are served well by this approach.

In chapter 2, we saw what happened when the board of Good Buddy Hospital approved the sale of real estate to a developer who wasn't even associated with the board. Let's change the facts a little and see what kind of trouble the board can cause itself by selling the property to one of its own members.

This time the board takes a little more care. It tells the administrator to get an appraisal and to make a written report on the proposed sale of the hospital's unneeded vacant land to Loyola Trust, a long-time director, civic leader, and highly motivated real estate tycoon. (The name of this director is entirely fictitious. If out there somewhere there is a hospital trustee named Loyola Trust, please accept the author's sincerest apologies.)

All of this is done, and at the next board meeting the sale is approved after Ms. Trust gives a little speech about how she intends to turn the land into a lovely subdivision that will be a credit to the community. She abstains from the vote and later makes millions from the transaction.

After suffering a series of devastating malpractice suits and settlements resulting from a careless credentialing decision, Good Buddy falls on hard times. Many former board members retire as their terms end, and an aggressive new board, dedicated to saving the hospital, emerges. As this board reviews the sorry history of the hospital's economic plunge, questions are raised concerning amounts paid to the hospital in the earlier land sale.

With regret, the new board determines that the terms of sale were unreasonably advantageous to Ms. Trust and injurious to the hospital corporation. It authorizes a suit against Ms. Trust alleging violation of her duty of loyalty to the corporation. The suit also names the other former directors, claiming that they knowingly allowed this breach of fiduciary duty to occur and that they also failed in their duty of care by allowing the corporation to be fleeced.

That's one way liability can turn up for the failure to place the interests of the hospital corporation above all others. There are many more. When directors engage in dealings with their corporations, the transactions should be so clearly advantageous to the corporation that they can withstand the closest and most skeptical scrutiny. Anything else begs trouble.

By the same token, when hospital attorneys, accountants, consultants, vendors, bankers, and others selling to the hospital serve on the board, they and the board enter into the shadow of risk. This is an area of vulnerability that deserves greater consideration, and it is dealt with again in chapter 7.

The Duty of Care

The duty of care is a common-law rule of common sense. Directors are expected to exercise at least the same degree of skill, care, and diligence in managing the affairs of the corporations they direct as reasonably prudent people would exercise in managing their own business affairs. In determining whether a director has met this obligation, courts apply a legal presumption known as the *business judgment rule*.

The Business Judgment Rule

Under the business judgment rule, it is presumed that the director has met the duty of care. With the presumption in play, it is up to any plaintiff to prove that the duty was breached—no easy task. The business judgment rule holds that a judgment or decision of a director—even if it turns out to be erroneous in retrospect—is presumed to meet the duty of care if three conditions have been met:

- The director obtained adequate information on which to base a reasonably informed judgment or decision about the matter under consideration.
- The director acted in good faith.
- The director believed that the decision made was in the best interest of the corporation.

This business judgment rule presumption is of tremendous importance to directors. It is based on and recognizes the fact that two equally informed and motivated people can arrive at different decisions regarding the matter before them. Under the rule, a director can be held liable to the corporation for breach of the duty of care for being sloppy or deceptive, but not merely for being wrong.

Let's take a closer look at each of the three conditions needed to activate the business judgment rule.

The director must obtain adequate information on which to make a reasonably informed judgment or decision about the matter under consideration.

Of the three conditions that you, as a loyal and trustworthy director, must meet, this is arguably the most important. It is also the one that most perplexes and confuses. What, after all, is "adequate information"?

It would be nice to have an easy formula to give you. But there is no little list that you can tuck into your pocket for the next board meeting. Determining what and how much information is adequate is a judgment call, and the nature of that judgment varies from situation to situation.

Nonetheless, a few generalizations can be made. Clearly, if a board has no information on which to base a decision, it runs the risk of having acted on the basis of "inadequate information."

Likewise, incomplete, unreliable, and suspect information may also be held to be inadequate. A hospital board that authorizes an expensive new program without any credible information on its economic feasibility would be hard-pressed to invoke the protection of the business judgment rule presumption if the board was later sued when the program (and the hospital) went belly up.

No, adequate information is the kind of information that our reasonably prudent person would demand before making a decision, and the "imagine you're on the witness stand" exercise described in chapter 2 may be the best way for a director to determine the presence or lack of adequate information in any given case.

The law does give boards one little boost in this area, however. Boards are generally entitled to rely on the reports and information provided to them by management. They are not generally expected to undertake independent study and ferret out information on their own.

Thus, when proposals are made to the board, are accompanied by studies and reports covering the financial, marketing, legal, quality, and other issues germane to a particular subject, and are conducted or made by individuals and firms thought to be competent in their fields, boards may rely on this information as being complete and accurate unless they have good reason to believe otherwise. Having *and using* this information, the board will generally be found to have armed itself with adequate information on which to base reasonably informed judgments.

What if a report to the board by management or a consultant working for the corporation draws conclusions or makes recommendations that are real laughers, completely unrealistic or unsupported by data or common experience? What if directors fail to read and question reports or fail to attend meetings and presentations at which information critical to a decision is made available?

The consequences should be clear. The director's information will probably be found to be inadequate if the decision is later alleged to have breached the duty of care. The presumption of the business judgment rule will be lost, and the director will have the duty to prove that the duty of care was met. Good luck!

The director must act in good faith.

This requirement sounds suspiciously like it belongs under the duty of loyalty standard discussed earlier and probably shows how strongly the duty of loyalty permeates every nook and cranny of the trustee's house. But we're talking about the duty of care and what it takes to qualify for the protection of the business judgment rule. What it takes is that you have to act in good faith.

Suppose that you're confronting a major issue for the hospital, say, the termination of an expensive contract with a hospital billing service. The administrator recommends a new vendor that will provide the same services at half the cost. The risk is that the new vendor is a small company and is relatively new to the field. All evidence points to its ability to perform, but if it runs into difficulties, the hospital will suffer.

It also happens that, unknown to the other trustees or the administrator, you are very good friends with the president of this proposed vendor. You don't have any economic interest in the company, but for many personal reasons you'd like to see your friend get the contract. At the board meeting you speak in favor of the contract change. You point out the benefit of receiving the services for less money, and you minimize the risk. By a split vote the board authorizes the administrator to make the change.

Doomsday scenario. The contract is too much for the new vendor to handle. Receivables go from 68 days to 112, and the hospital has to borrow money to meet its payroll. A suit is brought charging that the directors who approved the contract breached their duty of care to the corporation. You seek the protection of the business judgment rule—after all, you and the other board members had adequate information on which to base an informed judgment, and at the time it looked as though your decision was in the best interest of the corporation.

What's missing here, though, is good faith. The other directors who followed your lead might have done so in good faith. If so, they will be protected by the business judgment rule.

In your case, however, the plaintiffs have learned of your ties to the president of the new company. They claim that you failed to act in good faith, that your judgment was clouded by other factors, and that you multiplied your sin by misleading a majority of the board into a bad and costly decision for which *you* should pay. For you there is no presumption that you met the duty of care. You'll have to prove it to the jury. Ouch!

The director must believe that the decision made was in the best interest of the corporation.

The reader may ask, "When do directors ever make decisions that they don't honestly believe are in the best interests of the corporation?" From the cases that make it to court, it would appear that this occasionally happens when the director's judgment is overwhelmed by personal greed. It might also happen when directors forget the focus of their duty and use their board positions to benefit a "constituency."

Where greed gets in the way of a director's judgment and results in a failure of the duty of care, there will almost inevitably be a simultaneous breach of the duty of loyalty. In any event, this third condition to invoking the protection of the business judgment rule presumption simply says, "If you're playing director for your own benefit, don't expect to get any help from the courts." Indeed, any director who is caught double-dealing in violation of the fiduciary duties described here will be susceptible to liability for damages suffered by the corporation.

What happens, though, when a director makes decisions on behalf of a "constituency," and these decisions ultimately harm the corporation? This question might arise where a director is considered to "represent" some group or faction, such as the medical staff, hospital employees, or certain community interests. It might also happen (especially in not-for-profit and public corporations) where directors are elected by a parent organization and are expected to do that organization's bidding.

Take Good Buddy Hospital, for example. After its terrible financial collapse and internecine fighting, it was taken under the sponsorship of a Catholic religious order. Following a well-established model, the order operated the hospital corporation as a separate not-for-profit entity. Under Good Buddy's new bylaws, the order named all of the trustees and retained a number of reserve powers ensuring its control over the organization and its assets.

Good Buddy's order sponsors a number of other hospitals and nursing homes as well, and its headquarters office oversees all of the institutions and supplies various corporate shared services. This system works pretty well, and there is one understanding that binds it all together: When corporate speaks, the sponsored institutions are expected to jump.

After recovering somewhat from its financial woes, a couple of interesting things happen at Good Buddy. Corporate imposes a substantial charge to Good Buddy that is intended to cover Good Buddy's share of the corporate office's costly operating overhead. Then corporate, acting through Good Buddy's chairperson, changes Good Buddy's administrator more or less overnight. Both of these actions take place without prior board consultation. The approval of the Good Buddy board is obtained after the fact.

Now Good Buddy Hospital has been through enough distress in these two brief chapters to sink most hospital ships, and, in fact, it does not suffer as a result of these two moves by the parent corporation. But suppose things had not turned out so nicely. Suppose that the "corporate allocation" charges to Good Buddy had blown its mainsail and broken its rudder. Suppose that the new administrator had turned Good Buddy into an *Exxon Valdez*. Where would the board of Good Buddy stand then on the duty-to-exercise-care issue?

The fact is that under the common law the board is responsible for its own conduct. The business judgment rule provides a nice presumption of meeting the duty of care if the three conditions described here are met. But this third one, that decisions must be made with the belief that they are in the best interests of the corporation, is often difficult to abide in organizations with a chain of control and willful parents.

It is more than just possible that trustees in these settings will find themselves feeling compelled from time to time to make decisions that they don't necessarily believe are in the best interests of their local hospital organizations.

When they do so, and if things turn out poorly and they are sued, they may find that they have lost the protection of the business judgment rule.

This reality is only dimly understood in the hospital field today. It is one that deserves some attention from both the boards of local hospitals and the organizations under whose sponsorship or control those hospitals operate.

This same condition for gaining the protection of the business judgment rule applies to directors who feel that they represent a particular constituency. Not that there is any harm in voicing parochial concerns and points of view during the course of board deliberations; this activity is fine and probably desirable. But directors who make their board decisions on the basis of what is best for their constituencies rather than what is best for the corporation make a big mistake. Both the duty of loyalty and the condition of the business judgment rule described here require that decisions be based on what the director believes is best for the hospital corporation.

Attacks on the Business Judgment Rule

The reader may wonder why the author has lavished such great attention on the business judgment rule. After all, this book was supposed to be an easy read, and the business judgment rule is kind of technical, isn't it? Yes, but it is also the traditional keystone to a director's defense of all but knowing or intentional injuries to the corporation. If you understand this, you can understand why there has been a director scare and why premiums for director and officer liability insurance occasionally go through the roof and coverage availability dries up.

Lawsuits charging responsible and upstanding directors with a breach of the duty of care used to be losers. They would cause some inconvenience, but they constituted little more than a nuisance. "So I made a mistake," the director would say. "It was a business judgment."

The business judgment rule established the legal presumption that the director had acted with care. On the witness stand the defendant director would say: "I think I made a reasonable inquiry into this matter. I'm satisfied that the critical questions were thought about and answered credibly. Based on what I knew, what I was told, and what I believed, I honestly think that the decision I made was a good one for the corporation. Yes, it lost the corporation a bundle, but at the time it seemed like the right thing to do." Case dismissed.

In 1985, however, the Supreme Court of the State of Delaware decided a case (*Smith v. Van Gorkom*) that held that the very responsible and upstanding directors of Trans Union Corporation were not entitled to the business judgment rule presumption that they had exercised their duty of care.[1] Many of America's largest business corporations are incorporated under the laws of the State of Delaware, and when the Delaware Supreme

Court speaks concerning corporate law, people listen. The opinion in *Van Gorkom* caused a tremor in the force that even Darth Vader might have felt.

The directors of Trans Union voted to approve its sale in a very brief special meeting called one Saturday morning. The price per share in this transaction, which you might imagine was of some interest to the shareholders, was arrived at in a fashion that some observers, including the court, concluded was casual at best.

The plaintiffs in this case challenged the use of the business judgment rule. They said that some or all of the three conditions needed to gain the protection of the rule had not been met. Principal among these was that the directors had not received or sought adequate information on which to form a reasonably educated business judgment. The court agreed and denied the defendants the protection of the rule. The defendants were thus left to prove that they had acted in a manner that met their duty of care to the corporation and thus to the shareholders. They lost, and they paid. Millions.

In the wake of this case, many commentators cried that the business judgment rule was dead, and insurers panicked. But that was a while ago. Today, things are different and more stable.

First of all, the business judgment rule is not dead. Despite all their savvy and know-how, the directors in *Van Gorkom* did a dumb thing by failing to ensure that any reasonable measures were taken to determine the value of the corporation. When you or I sell our homes and we're smart, we get a couple of independent market appraisals before we set the price. The directors in *Van Gorkom* didn't do that, or anything like that, and the court therefore concluded that they didn't satisfy the conditions for application of the business judgment rule.

Later, insurance prices came back down and availability went back up, indicating that the panic was over for a while.

The Need to Keep Informed

What, then, is the message to the reader of this book? It's this: Assuming good faith and loyalty to the corporation, if you're a director of a hospital corporation you must actively seek to inform yourself regarding matters coming to your attention. Blind and unquestioning reliance on the recommendations and opinions of others is not sufficient.

Directors are not expected to recreate the work of management, committees, or consultants, but they are expected to be aware of laws and legal standards that apply to issues under consideration. They are expected to attend meetings at which information is provided, read reports directed to their attention, and verify that those to whom they have delegated functions have performed with reasonable competence and credibility.

Directors are expected to question obvious omissions, inconsistencies, and inaccuracies. They are also expected to be familiar with, and abide by, the standards and requirements contained in the articles of incorporation, corporate bylaws, medical staff bylaws, and formal policies of the organization. Failure in this regard leaves the director without a reasonable factual basis for decision making. Without such a basis a director is hard-pressed to justify a decision—especially one that is ultimately harmful to the corporation.

Thus, the duty of care is the duty of hard work. Failure to comply with this duty can leave the director liable to the corporation for the damages it has suffered as a result of the director's malfeasance.

The Duty of Obedience

The duty of obedience sounds like something that comes out of dog training school or what we tell our children. For human, adult corporate directors, however, it is simply the duty to *obey* the law. *The law* in this case includes a lot: state statutes governing corporations, the corporation's articles of incorporation and bylaws, and a broad range of other state and federal laws governing the conduct of businesses and individuals.

State Corporation Laws Prohibiting Specific Acts

The corporation laws of the various states set forth instances in which directors can be held liable to the corporation and to third parties. For example, loans by a not-for-profit corporation to officers and directors are often prohibited by state law. In these cases, directors who approve such loans can be held liable for their payment. Also, in many states, directors are liable to the corporation for unauthorized distribution of corporate assets and liable to creditors for failing to notify them of the dissolution of the corporation or for carrying on business in the corporation's name after dissolution.

Other State Corporation Laws

State corporation statutes describe the acts in which corporations may engage and place limits on the authority of the board of directors. They also set forth procedures that must be followed for many important corporate actions, such as electing officers and directors, amending articles of incorporation and bylaws, merging with other corporations, and disposing of corporate assets.

In the case of business and not-for-profit corporations, the laws regarding corporate and director authority usually provide great latitude. The corporation can usually undertake all legal activities necessary to carry out its stated purpose, and directors are usually authorized to do all of the things reasonably related to the management of the corporation. In public corporations, however, the scope of the corporation's and the board's authority is typically more limited and detailed.

Actions taken by corporations and their boards that exceed the limits of statutory authority or that violate specific statutory requirements are *ultra vires,* or beyond the law, and can be voided. Directors who are responsible for allowing such *ultra vires* acts to take place can sometimes be held liable to the corporation and to third parties for the injuries that such acts may have occasioned.

Let's illustrate these points with an example. Titanic Medical Center is a freestanding, inner-city hospital that serves the poor. It is a not-for-profit, membership corporation. Most of its members are pastors from local churches. Because of the financial difficulties of operating the hospital and the need to tap corporations for gifts, however, over the years the members have elected outsiders to the board, primarily executives of some of the city's major companies.

The care for over 90 percent of Titanic's patients is paid for by Medicare and Medicaid, and underpayment by these payers has resulted in continued operating losses. Eventually the center falls into serious debt, and the board sees no way to turn things around.

A for-profit group approaches Titanic's board with an offer to buy the facility for conversion into a psychiatric hospital. The board is not happy about this approach, but the sale appears to be its only viable option. Independent appraisals of the hospital's assets are made, and the board authorizes the sale at a fair price. After the closing, the proceeds from the sale are used to pay off Titanic's outstanding debts, and work commences on the dissolution of the corporation.

This is not a happy picture, and it gets worse. In the state where Titanic is incorporated, the corporation law requires that "the sale of all or substantially all of the assets of the corporation shall be subject to the approval of the members of the corporation, if any members there shall be."

Well, Titanic has lots of members, and their approval of the sale transaction was never sought or obtained. In fact, those members are furious about the sale and closing of the only general hospital serving the area. The members enlist the involvement of the state's attorney general, and a successful suit is brought to void the sale of the hospital as an *ultra vires* act.

What happens next is the thing that directors' nightmares are made of. After the hospital is deeded back to Titanic Medical Center Corporation (whose board has been replaced under court order), the buyer seeks to regain the funds it paid. Most of these, of course, have been paid to the medical center's former creditors. Ultimately, the buyer sues the medical center and its former board members for restitution of the illegally acquired funds, and the new board of Titanic sues the former board, seeking damages for the *ultra vires* act and the former board's violation of its duty of care.

The whole episode is played up big by the local press with headlines reading: "Trustees Sink Titanic!" The cases are settled, and the former board members, through their director and officer (D&O) liability insurance, pay.

The next year, D&O coverage for hospital boards across the country doubles in cost and availability dries up.

This is a fictitious case, but it shows why it is important that directors obey the requirements of the law under which their corporation is organized. It also is interesting to note that, as in the example above, liability can arise for *ultra vires* acts even though no violation was intended. Indeed, such unintentional *ultra vires* acts often have much in common with violations of the duty of care, another area in which intent is not a factor.

More often, however, *ultra vires* activities have an element of willfulness in them, and nowhere is this as prevalent as in struggles for control of the corporation. These struggles may involve violations of both state statutes and corporate documents concerning the vehicles of control — changes to articles of incorporation and bylaws, the election of corporate directors and officers, and others.

Corporate Documents

Within the context and limits of state laws, corporations make their own specific rules. These are found in their articles of incorporation and corporate bylaws. The articles of incorporation follow a pattern required by state statute. They are filed, approved, and recorded with a state official, typically the secretary of state. Any amendments to the articles of incorporation must also be filed, approved, and recorded.

The bylaws of the corporation are usually internal to the organization. Although they are subordinate to the state corporation laws and the articles of incorporation, in terms of establishing rules for the activities and governance of the corporation, they are every bit as important.

In business and not-for-profit corporations the composition of the board, requirements for board membership, methods for election, plurality requirements, and similar provisions are stated in the articles or bylaws or in both. Rules for amending the articles and bylaws are also found in these documents. (For public corporations these details are usually contained in state statutes.) Where members or shareholders have reserve powers in excess of those contained in statutory law, these are likewise stated in the corporate documents.

All of this forms a complex set of rules, a sort of lawyers' playground, that lend themselves to varying interpretations or outright violations when different factions vie for control of the corporation. Violations of these corporate rules by the corporation and its directors are *ultra vires* and invite attack in the form of litigation and possible director liability.

When such suits arise, they are often among the corporate directors and officers themselves, and they tend to be pretty acrimonious. In addition to one faction charging the other with unauthorized (and therefore voidable) corporate acts, frequently there are also charges of defamation and of breaches of the duties of loyalty and care. These suits are mean and dirty and make up a large percentage of the successful director litigation that takes place.

The Internal Revenue Code

The federal Internal Revenue Code holds corporate directors personally liable in certain instances in which the corporation has failed to pay over payroll taxes that have been withheld from employees. Fortunately, state and federal laws don't usually hold directors accountable for this level of operational detail, and in viable organizations it is unlikely that directors will have to spend much time worrying about this particular exposure.

But the managers of failing organizations sometimes view employee withholdings as a source of cash with which to pay C.O.D. vendors and to keep the business running. This is a form of theft, and the message from Congress is that the directors of the corporation are expected to keep the practice from occurring.

Criminal and Civil Wrongful Acts

Directors are personally responsible and liable for their own criminal conduct. If a director, acting solely or in concert with other directors, officers, or employees, steals or embezzles from the corporation or engages in illegal insider trading or other such activities, the punishment can be fines and imprisonment. In addition, the director will be liable to the corporation for the injury it has suffered.

If directors knowingly act to cause the corporation to engage in criminal acts, the liability can be direct and personal as well. This is as it should be, for public policy could not in good conscience allow directors to play at will and without rules behind the fictitious and artificial veil of the corporation that the state itself has authorized and empowered.

Suppose, for example, that the directors of a hospital corporation instructed management to circumvent certificate-of-need laws in order to build a new facility or to dump hazardous infectious wastes rather than contract and pay for lawful disposal or to implement or maintain clearly illegal discriminatory practices in the hiring or treatment of employees. The criminal liability for these acts would lead to the directors, and they could be prosecuted. Fines and penalties levied against the hospital corporation could, in turn, be recouped from the guilty directors as a result of their breach of duty to the corporation.

Consider as an example this news squib, even though it doesn't involve a hospital transaction:

SUNDSTRAND SETTLES WITH HOLDERS

Sundstrand Corp. said its insurance companies agreed to pay $15 million to settle shareholder litigation against some current and former officers and directors of the Rockford-based defense contractor, arising out of its 1988 guilty plea to defense fraud charges. Sundstrand paid a then-record $115 million to settle the government's procurement fraud charges. Shareholders in turn sued officers and directors for the damage to the company. Harry C. Stonecipher, president and chief executive, said: "This development puts the company's past difficulties squarely behind it."[2]

That this kind of activity happens so seldom in the hospital arena is a credit to the integrity of the directors who sit on hospital boards.

Noncriminal but tortious acts can also result in personal liability for directors. Defamation of character, wrongful interference with contract, retaliatory employee discharge, and similar actions are samples of conduct that might result in director liability to a third person.

Say, for example, that during the course of reappointing physicians to the medical staff a director singles out one of the doctors and tells the other directors: "That incompetent SOB shouldn't be permitted to care for rabid dogs. Anyone who allows that doctor to provide care runs a good risk of ending up in a funeral parlor." Not exactly flattering words. Whether or not the doctor is reappointed, when this description makes the rounds, the accusing director may find himself or herself served with a legal summons and complaint alleging slander. The boardroom provides very little protection for what may be the reckless defamation of a person's good name and reputation.

Director action resulting in the hospital corporation's termination of a contract might also result in a claim or suit naming members of the board. Suppose, for example, that for unsavory reasons of their own a group of directors prevail on the administrator to end a service or a supply contract. The vendor might very well charge that the personal actions of the directors in the undertaking constituted a tortious interference with the contractual relationship and that the directors should be held personally liable for the damages the vendor suffered as a result. Such suits do arise occasionally, and they are sometimes brought by contracting physicians and employees as well. If the plaintiffs can prove their cases, directors won't be shielded by the corporation or the director role.

A third area of exposure to tortious liability is retaliatory discharge. In one case, suppose that an employee of the hospital files a discrimination suit against the corporation and the suit so angers the board of directors that the board orders the administrator to fire the employee immediately.

In another case, suppose that an employee learns that the hospital managers have been involved in illegal conduct, such as bribing a public official or burning hazardous waste in the wee hours of the night. The employee informs the board about the conduct and adds that if action is not taken, the matter will be reported to the appropriate government enforcement authorities. Being so forced, the board grudgingly takes the necessary action to stop and report the illegal activities. Later, though, the board urges the administrator to "get rid of that unloyal employee who caused us all the trouble by blowing the whistle." In these instances, the individual directors might find themselves personally on the defendant end of a lawsuit, and they might very well lose.

These and similar actions have a couple of things in common. They all involve acts that might be found to be civil wrongs in many states, and they all involve direct action and participation by members of the board. They have another common thread as well. All may entitle a successful plaintiff to punitive damages in addition to the actual damages the plaintiff has suffered. Sometimes the actual damages are relatively small, but the punitive damages run into the millions.

Some Troubling Questions about Hospital Director Liability

It's not hard to understand why directors face exposure to personal liability in the instances cited in the preceding sections. In every instance (save potential liability to the tax person), directors are front stage and center. They alone control their conduct, and it is logical that they should be responsible for its consequences.

But what about criminal and civil wrongful conduct where the board did not play a role or where its role was passive at most? Let's take an illustration on the criminal side.

Suppose that in order to recruit doctors and increase hospital admissions the administrator at Stichem Community Hospital undertook an aggressive program of monetary incentives. Everything the administrator did was so patently illegal under the federal Medicare fraud and abuse statutes that we can call the incumbent a felon without any qualms or doubts. Some new doctors were drawn to Stichem, and they and a few of the doctors already on staff started admitting heavily to the hospital. The hospital's census underwent a noticeable improvement, and so did the monthly financial statement.

Eventually, the administrator was indicted in federal court, and the hospital faced heavy fines and loss of Medicare and Medicaid participation. The board never had any idea of what was going on. Is there a likelihood of federal prosecution or other liability for the board of directors in this scenario?

Let's suppose further that the administrator had on several occasions sought and received authorization from the board to spend very large sums of money on "physician incentives." The administrator seemed to be getting results, and the board always went along with these requests without inquiring into their specific use or legality. Is the board's liability and criminal exposure increased by this activity?

Then let's suppose that one of the board members heard that the administrator was paying physicians cash for each admission made to the hospital. Many physicians resented this practice, and it was said that it violated the law. The director passed the word along to the other trustees, but no one raised the issue with the administrator or at a board meeting. Any change yet in exposure?

Finally, let's suppose that this entire program and its illegality were discussed fully by the board and the administrator. The program yielded great results and the hospital was no longer insolvent. The board, in effect, told the administrator, "Keep up the good work, but if you get caught, we never knew what you were doing." Have the directors gone too far to escape criminal or other liability?

The answer to this final question is probably yes. The answers to the questions raised along the way are less certain. At what point should the trustees have delved into the administrator's incentive program to determine its propriety? Learning of its impropriety, what should the directors have done? These are all difficult questions, but as the scrutiny of hospitals increases and accountability of directors is widened, the ability of hospital directors to say, "Gee, I didn't know any of that was going on," and get away with it is sure to decrease.

Equally troubling questions arise on the civil liability side of the equation. Take, for example, Stichem Community Hospital's ailing open-heart surgery program. The cardiac surgeons in charge of the program keep working at perfecting their techniques, but the patients keep leaving the operating room dead. The mortality rate for the program hovers around 25 percent, alarmingly above the national average. And this is only the tip of the iceberg. The directors of Stichem know that this program along with many others has an abysmal quality rating and has come apart at the seams, and yet they do nothing to mend the tear.

And look at Stichem's medical staff credentialing process. Every misfit and reject licensed to practice medicine can find a home at Stichem Community Hospital. The credentialing process is so full of holes that over a short period of time two unlicensed individuals managed to gain membership with full clinical privileges in their fantasy specialties. The board knows vaguely that there have been staff quality problems and once asked the administrator and medical chief of staff what could be done. "All hospitals have these kinds of problems," they were told, "and our credentialing could stand up anywhere." This was sort of a confusing area, and so the board decided to leave it alone.

Now, much earlier, we learned that boards can't be sued by the public for the negligence of the hospital or members of its medical staff. As they undertake their acts and deliberations, the directors have a duty to the hospital corporation. But if boards know or should know about severe and life-threatening problems or other corporate activities that create a menace and threat to the community and fail to do anything about them, can this separation from liability provided by the law be maintained? This is a question that will be decided in the courts. The best policy for directors is to act as though it's already been decided in favor of the public through broader board liability.

Special Standards for Hospital Directors

Duty of loyalty, duty of care, and duty of obedience—these are the legally recognized duties that apply to directors in every corporate setting, within and outside the hospital field. The breach of these duties can result in liability. There are other legal rules and standards that apply solely to hospital directors, however, and the duties of care and of obedience obligate hospital directors to be familiar with these standards and to meet them as they govern their hospital organizations.

State Standards

A survey of the special state-mandated responsibilities of hospital directors would be too lengthy for this book, but each director should gain knowledge of whatever statutory and regulatory standards may apply to hospital boards in the hospital's jurisdiction. Failure of directors to be cognizant of these standards and to employ reasonable means to meet them could constitute a violation of the duties of care and obedience.

Occasionally, a state's rules for hospital governance are found in statutes. This is especially true for public hospitals, such as county and district hospitals, authorized by special laws. Most often, however, the standards are contained in regulations adopted by the state department in charge of public health or hospital licensing.

The most important of these state standards concerning governance relate to policy, management, medical staff affairs, and quality assurance matters. One state prescribes these standards as follows:

- For each hospital there shall be a governing authority responsible for its organization, management, control, and operations, including appointment of the medical staff.
- The board shall employ a competent executive officer or administrator and vest that person with the authority to carry out its policies.
- The board shall ensure employment of competent, well-qualified personnel in adequate numbers to carry out the functions of the hospital.

- The board shall be responsible for the maintenance of standards of professional work in the hospital and shall require that the medical staff function competently. Clinical audits shall be performed by the medical staff and reviewed by a committee of the governing authority and medical staff.

At this point the reader who is a hospital director might be wondering whether the state standards for governance in the state in which the hospital is licensed have ever been presented to and reviewed by the board of the director's hospital. It's a good bet that the answer is no, at least not within recent memory.

So think again about taking the witness stand and responding to this swipe in your own director liability suit: "Certainly you don't mean to tell the ladies and gentlemen of the jury that you served on the board of [your] hospital for three and one-half years and never sought to educate yourself concerning the most basic and fundamental rules of hospital governance promulgated by the public health officials of this state?"

In fact, directors probably run very little risk of ever being sued for their failure to read and be familiar with the standards for governance in their states. But in other director suits alleging a breach of the duty of care or a breach of the duty of obedience, a failure in this regard is another three-penny nail in the coffin. It makes the director look dumb and negligent.

More important, these standards can provide directors with important guidance concerning some of the priorities of the board. If state public health officials have thought long and hard to come up with a laundry list of what the people in charge of hospital governance should be doing, directors can be thankful and can use the list to figure out just what is important. Most states think that the quality of the medical staff and the quality of hospital services are among the most important things governance can concern itself with.

Joint Commission Standards

No less important than the state standards for hospital governance are the standards adopted by the Joint Commission on Accreditation of Healthcare Organizations. These standards are more comprehensive than those found in many states, and in hospitals with Joint Commission accreditation, they have much the same force as law. Most hospitals without such accreditation are covered by federal Medicare rules of participation, which parallel many aspects of the Joint Commission standards.

The Joint Commission standards are contained in the *Accreditation Manual for Hospitals,* which is updated and reprinted every year. One suspects, however, that the standards pertaining to the organization and function of the hospital governing body (as the Joint Commission likes to refer to hospital boards of directors) only seldom leave the administrator's bookshelf to find their way to the directors.

This is not good. Directors should pay the same heed to these standards as to state standards for governance, and for the same reasons.

The Joint Commission's standards are so concise that an attempt to summarize them is probably counterproductive. It is simply better that hospital directors read them completely at least once a year.

What is important to communicate here, however, is that the Joint Commission standards hold hospital boards responsible for most important aspects of hospital management and require that detailed activities be performed and documented by the board. A copy of the 1991 accreditation standards for hospital governing bodies is reprinted with the permission of the Joint Commission as appendix A in this book.

Final Words on the Legal Duties of Directors

Earlier, it was said that the duty of care is the duty of hard work, and you can see why. But hard work, loyalty, and integrity are the recognized stock-in-trade of so many American hospital directors and of so many who might one day serve on hospital boards. By exercising these traits—by not leaving good sense and judgment behind when hospital business is at hand—the directors of hospitals of every kind will provide themselves with strong armor against the threat of liability.

And it is important to know that society is not somehow out to get the directors of corporations. Plaintiffs' counsels may concoct clever and appealing new theories of liability, and judges may be slow to turn them away, but at the same time legislators around the country have heeded a call for more statutory protection for directors of corporations of all kinds and in some cases have been especially kind to the directors of hospitals. These protections and others are described in chapter 4.

☐ *References*

1. Smith v. Van Gorkom, 488 A.2d 858.
2. *Chicago Tribune,* Business Section, Aug. 10, 1990, p. 1.

Chapter 4

The "Three Eyes": Immunity, Indemnity, and Insurance

Honest, loyal, and conscientious work is the best means of ensuring that a hospital director is never the victim of personal liability resulting from participation in governance. It is no guarantee, however, that a director will never be made subject to a claim.

For this reason, most states now afford directors additional protections aimed at preventing lawsuits or saving directors from actual financial loss. These aids through the thicket of potential liability can be thought of as the "three eyes": immunity, indemnity, and insurance.

Immunity

If you were a monarch with absolute power, you could do anything you wanted and no one could sue you. You could become a despot. People might be tempted to do something worse than sue you, but court action to stop, punish, or recover damages for your terrible deeds would be out of the question. You would be protected by sovereign immunity, and you could laugh away the consequences of your dastardly acts. This is real immunity in action.

Immunity for directors of corporations is something else. First of all, in order for directors to gain protection from lawsuits, there must be legislative action in the form of enabling legislation granting the immunity or limiting liability. Second, these enabling laws almost never protect criminal or other intentionally wrongful acts. Third, when such grants are made, they typically are narrowly drawn and subject to conditions and limitations. When the statutes granting director immunity are considered in the courts, they are strictly construed. Our system of justice does not take kindly to laws that limit personal accountability for wrongful behavior.

Thus, the first "eye"—immunity—may not provide great comfort to all hospital directors in all cases. Still, from the director's point of view, some immunity is better than none at all, and it's worth taking a look at the level of protection provided by statutes that limit liability.

Categories of Statutes

Statutes providing directors with immunity or otherwise limiting director liability fall into three broad categories: state corporation laws, state laws dealing with medical staff credentialing, and the federal Health Care Quality Improvement Act of 1986. This business of categorization gets a little dry, but it is a helpful way of understanding and remembering the nature of protection the law can afford.

Corporation Statutes

After the *Smith v. Van Gorkom*[1] case (which we discussed in chapter 3), and the director and officer liability insurance crisis that followed *Van Gorkom,* many states amended their corporation laws to erect new barriers to director liability. These actions were taken with the single avowed purpose of enhancing corporate governance by limiting the spectre of director liability.

The approaches of these statutes vary widely among business, not-for-profit, and public corporations, but they all have one thing in common: They make it more difficult to sue directors for breaches of the *duty of care*. Appropriately, they do little or nothing to limit liability for breaches of the duties of loyalty and obedience.

In the business corporation sphere, at least 33 states have adopted statutes to limit the liability of corporate directors. Many jurisdictions have adopted the approach taken in Delaware: Shareholders may amend the articles of incorporation of the company to foreclose suits against directors and officers by shareholders or the corporation when a breach of the duty of care is at issue. Other states have enacted self-executing statutes, which provide this new level of protection without the need for shareholder action. Some states have also established liability caps covering almost all derivative suits against directors.[2]

Immunity and other liability limitation statutes enacted to cover not-for-profit and public hospitals are almost all self-executing. Currently, at least 46 jurisdictions have laws on their books providing some form of liability protection for trustees of private, not-for-profit hospitals. These jurisdictions are listed in figure 4-1, and a summary of these state laws is provided in appendix B.

Some of these laws limiting the liability of trustees of not-for-profit and public corporations may provide a greater reach of protection than the laws

Figure 4-1. Jurisdictions with Corporation Laws Providing Some Form of Immunity for the Directors of Private, Not-for-Profit Hospital Corporations*

Alabama	Kansas	Nevada	Rhode Island
Arkansas	Kentucky	New Hampshire	South Carolina
California	Louisiana	New Jersey	South Dakota
Colorado	Maine	New Mexico	Tennessee
Delaware	Maryland	New York	Texas
Florida	Massachusetts	North Carolina	Utah
Georgia	Michigan	North Dakota	Vermont
Hawaii	Minnesota	Ohio	Washington
Idaho	Mississippi	Oklahoma	West Virginia
Illinois	Missouri	Oregon	Wisconsin
Indiana	Montana	Pennsylvania	Wyoming
Iowa	Nebraska		

*A listing of statutory citations is provided in appendix B.

in the business corporation sector. Although the for-profit corporation laws are aimed at thwarting shareholder and corporate suits against directors, many statutes in the nonprofit arena would seem to preclude suits brought by anyone, including members of the general public, as long as the conditions contained in the statutes are met.

But there are conditions. Many of them are reasonable and understandable; others raise questions and doubts that ultimately will be decided in the courts. Depending on the state, directors of nonprofit hospitals may not be protected by immunity legislation when there are allegations of gross negligence, intentional harm, willful or wanton misconduct, or intentional tortious conduct. In many states, only uncompensated trustees are protected. Figure 4-2 shows the main conditions and limitations.

The immunity provision found in the Illinois Not for Profit Corporation Act is a good example of what these protective statutes do and fail to do. This entire law was revised in 1986 and incorporated a fairly sweeping limitation on director liability:

> No director or officer serving *without compensation,* other than reimbursement for actual expenses, of a corporation organized under this [Illinois Not for Profit Corporation] Act and exempt, or qualified for exemption, from taxation pursuant to Section 501(c) of the Internal Revenue Code of 1986, as amended, shall be liable, and no cause of action may be brought, for damages *resulting from the exercise of judgment or discretion* in connection with the duties or responsibilities of such director or officer *unless the act or omission involved willful or wanton conduct.* [Emphasis added.][3]

Figure 4-2. Principal Conditions to and Limitations on Immunity for Directors of Private, Not-for-Profit Hospital Corporations

Must be uncompensated director: Alabama, California, Colorado, Delaware, Georgia, Hawaii, Idaho, Illinois, Indiana, Kentucky, Louisiana, Maine, Minnesota, Missouri, Nebraska, New Hampshire, New Jersey, New York, North Carolina, North Dakota, Oklahoma, Rhode Island, South Carolina, South Dakota, Vermont, West Virginia

Require showing of good faith: California, Idaho, Kansas, Kentucky, Louisiana, New Hampshire, North Carolina, North Dakota, Oklahoma, South Dakota, Texas, Vermont

No protection in discrimination matters: California

Willful and wanton conduct excluded: Alabama, Arkansas, California, Colorado, Delaware, Florida, Georgia, Iowa, Idaho, Illinois, Kansas, Kentucky, Louisiana, Maryland, Michigan, Minnesota, Missouri, Montana, Nebraska, Nevada, New Hampshire, New Jersey, New Mexico, New York, North Carolina, North Dakota, Oklahoma, Pennsylvania, Rhode Island, South Carolina, South Dakota, Tennessee, Texas, Vermont, Washington, Wisconsin

Gross negligence excluded: Alabama, Arkansas, California, Delaware, Georgia, Hawaii, Maryland, Michigan, Missouri, New Jersey, New York, North Carolina, North Dakota, Oklahoma, South Carolina, Tennessee, Texas, Vermont, West Virginia

Reckless acts excluded: California, Florida, New Mexico, New York, Pennsylvania, South Carolina, Texas

---

There is not much mystery in this statute. It protects directors of most Illinois not-for-profit hospitals against claims brought in Illinois courts by, or in the name of, the corporation and claims by members of the general public as long as three conditions are met.

First, a director must serve without compensation other than reimbursement for actual expenses. One might quibble over the meaning of *compensation*—whether a free meal served in connection with a board meeting, for instance, or the provision of first-class rooms, meals, and recreation at an off-site board retreat constitutes compensation. Lacking any court interpretation, it is probably a safe bet that such common and reasonable services provided by the hospital corporation in connection with board activities would not breach this condition.

Other board perquisites, such as free or discounted hospital care, however, might be viewed as compensation. Also, reimbursement for travel and other expenses to distant and lavish resorts for activities and programs of questionable applicability to board performance might cause problems. The point to bear in mind is that in enacting this provision the legislature sought to give protection to a deserving class of volunteer directors, and abuses of this protection are not likely to be tolerated by the courts.

Second, the provision protects only the acts involving the business judgment and discretion of directors. In its essence, the provision serves to codify and strengthen the protection traditionally applied to directors under the common-law business judgment rule. You will recall that the business judgment rule establishes a presumption that directors have met the duty of care when they have obtained adequate information, acted in good faith, and believed that a decision was in the best interest of the corporation. This statutory provision changes the presumption, which is susceptible to rebuttal by a plaintiff, into a nonrebuttable legal rule that the duty of care has been met in all instances.

Third, however, this protection does not apply to director acts or omissions that involve "willful or wanton conduct." As mentioned earlier, in some states this holdback of protection occurs as well where there are allegations of gross negligence, intentional harm, or intentional tortious conduct on the part of directors.

These terms are not always defined in the statutes, and where this is the case, directors must look to the common law for guidance. In the Illinois statute, however, the term *willful or wanton conduct* is clearly defined and generally will satisfy most directors that they are unlikely to stray from the protection of the immunity provision:

> As used in this Section "willful or wanton conduct" means a course of action which shows an actual or deliberate intention to cause harm or which, if not intentional, shows an utter indifference to or conscious disregard for the safety of others or their property.[4]

Thus, under the Illinois law, in order for a plaintiff to avoid dismissal of a suit for damages against directors, there must be an allegation of one or more of the following:

- The organization does not qualify for exemption under Section 501(c) of the Internal Revenue Code.
- The defendant directors receive compensation for their services.
- The directors' acts or omissions giving rise to damages were intended to cause harm.
- The directors' acts or omissions giving rise to damages showed an utter indifference to, or conscious disregard for, the safety of others or their property.

The reader will no doubt recognize intuitively that in most American hospital settings this would be a sizable burden for a plaintiff to overcome. The vast majority of U.S. hospitals are recognized as tax-exempt and are served by volunteers who donate their time without compensation. Most people would be hard-pressed to cite an instance in which hospital directors acted with the intent of causing harm to their hospital corporation or to any other person or thing. Thus, state attorneys general, successor boards, aggrieved doctors, former employees, and most other potential plaintiffs face an uphill battle when they contemplate director suits in states with immunity statutes like that in Illinois.

If there is a catch, it is in the fourth bullet—the one dealing with "utter indifference to, or conscious disregard for, the safety of others or their property": taking action, allowing action to take place, or failing to take needed action without troubling oneself regarding the consequences. The immunity statute may allow directors to be sloppy and negligent, but it does not protect them when they knowingly ignore problems or take actions they know can result in harm to others and their property, and such harm does, in fact, occur.

In chapter 3, for example, we discussed two problems at Stichem Community Hospital. One involved an open-heart surgery program with an amazingly high mortality rate, and the other involved a medical staff credentialing process that simply didn't work. The board of Stichem was aware of both problems, but rather than delve into them and ensure that corrective steps were taken, it let them slide. As a result, patients were maimed and killed. The Stichem directors would not find much comfort in typical director immunity statutes like the one described because they acted (or failed to act) with utter indifference to, and conscious disregard for, the safety of others.

Whether the directors could be brought to task by injured patients or the survivors of the dead is still doubtful. But after those people sue the hospital corporation into bankruptcy, successor boards or the state attorney general would have a clear right to sue and collect from the old directors on behalf of the hospital. Immunity statutes aren't meant to protect directors who are aggressively uncaring.

State Medical Staff Credentialing Immunity Laws

Another form of state statutory immunity increasingly in favor relates to director liability in the instance of credentialing and other quality assurance decisions. Busy state hospital associations are increasingly successful in getting state legislatures to buy in to the notion that hospitals and their boards should be shielded from liability in this area if they are to play a tough and proactive role in keeping troublesome practitioners out of hospitals. A list of the jurisdictions providing some form of immunity to hospital directors in connection with credentialing and other peer review activities is shown in figure 4-3.

These enabling laws serve to bar or limit monetary damages against hospitals and their boards when a suit is brought by a practitioner who has been denied medical staff membership or who has been subject to corrective action. We'll look at a statute from Illinois again because it is one that is particularly generous in the protection it provides and has held up under the scrutiny of the state's appellate courts:

> No hospital and no individual who is a member, agent, or employee of a hospital, hospital medical staff, hospital administrative staff, or *hospital governing board* shall be liable for *civil damages* as a result

Figure 4-3. Jurisdictions That Provide Some Level of Immunity from Liability for Members of Medical Peer Review Committees*

Alabama	Illinois	Missouri	Pennsylvania
Alaska	Indiana	Montana	Rhode Island
Arizona	Iowa	Nebraska	South Carolina
Arkansas	Kansas	Nevada	South Dakota
California	Kentucky	New Hampshire	Tennessee
Colorado	Louisiana	New Jersey	Texas
Delaware	Maine	New Mexico	Utah
District of Columbia	Maryland	New York	Vermont
Florida	Massachusetts	North Carolina	Washington
Georgia	Michigan	North Dakota	West Virginia
Hawaii	Minnesota	Ohio	Wisconsin
Idaho	Mississippi	Oklahoma	Wyoming

*A listing of statutory citations is provided in appendix C.

of the acts, omissions, decisions, or any other conduct of a medical utilization committee, medical review committee, patient care audit committee, medical care evaluation committee, quality review committee, credentials committee, peer review committee, or any other committee whose purpose, directly or indirectly, is internal quality control or medical study to reduce morbidity or mortality, or for improving patient care within a hospital, or the improving or benefiting of patient care and treatment, whether within a hospital or not, or for the purpose of professional discipline. Nothing in this Section shall relieve any individual or hospital from liability arising from treatment of a patient. [Emphasis added.][5]

This statute, which protects for-profit, not-for-profit, and public hospitals, is like a steel door. Under its provisions, an aggrieved physician can sue the hospital and can attempt to sue the board, but there can be no award of damages. The effect of the statute has been to foreclose all but suits for injunctive relief to correct alleged failures to follow procedures set forth in medical staff bylaws. There is little reason to name hospital directors in this type of suit.

Not all state statutes are as sweeping as the one from Illinois. Many require a showing of good faith before any statutory protection can be invoked. Others stop short of providing immunity from liability in cases where malicious or other activity intended to cause harm to the practitioner who brings suit has been alleged.

Federal Health Care Quality Improvement Act

One thing that state director immunity laws can't protect against is suits that are based on federal law and brought in federal courts. Foremost among these are civil antitrust suits based on alleged violations of federal laws. These suits are expensive to defend against and can result in substantial damage verdicts when the plaintiff prevails. Ever since the U.S. Supreme Court ruled in the 1970s that hospitals were subject to certain federal antitrust laws, antitrust suits against hospitals and their directors have mounted in frequency.

Enter the Health Care Quality Assurance Act of 1986. This strange law of ambiguous origin holds itself out as offering hospitals and their boards protection from federal antitrust civil liability, as well as state civil liability in certain cases. This protection may be more illusory than real, but because the law deals with federal questions that cannot be treated under state law and also provides a measure of immunity in states that have not made their own immunity grants, it bears a moment of study.

Interest in regaining protection from federal antitrust liability reached its zenith after the U.S. Supreme Court in 1988 upheld a District Court finding that doctors on a hospital medical staff credentials committee had conspired to remove a competing doctor from the medical staff of an Astoria, Oregon, hospital *(Patrick v. Burget)*.[6] The $2.2 million judgment against the doctors was not covered by director and officer liability insurance, and some of the defendants were said to have been ruined financially. Although this judgment caused many doctors, hospitals, and hospital boards to seek the refuge of the Health Care Quality Improvement Act, it is important to realize that the act was never intended to authorize or protect the kind of illegal behavior that the court found in *Patrick*.

The act seeks to promote professional review activities by providing limited immunity to peer review activities. In the hospital setting the law establishes a presumption that a hospital, directors, and others have acted within the law in taking adverse credentialing and other quality assurance actions vis-à-vis a practitioner. As always, a number of conditions must be met before the presumption of innocence can be invoked by the defendants. Also, the immunity provided by the act does not extend to civil rights actions, suits seeking injunctive relief, or enforcement actions brought by the United States or state attorneys general.

The preconditions to invoking the immunity of the act are numerous. To obtain the immunity, the professional review action must be taken in the *reasonable belief* that the action was in the furtherance of high-quality health care. Meeting this requirement requires good faith and an unknown level of substantive due process. Even when the other conditions of the act are met, if it appears that an adverse credentialing decision was not justified by the facts or that it was motivated by other than a good-faith belief that it was necessary for high-quality care, the *reasonable belief* requirement will not have been met and the protection of the act will have been lost.

The act also requires that *adequate notice and hearing procedures* must be given to the practitioner involved, and it sets forth a series of demanding notice and hearing procedures that meet Congress's notion of what is fair and adequate. A hospital is free to follow other notice and hearing procedures it believes to be "fair" under the circumstances, but using procedures different from those identified in the act invites an aggrieved practitioner to challenge them as "unfair." This can be dangerous because a successful challenge invalidates the act's immunity.

In order to meet the adequate notice and hearing requirements conclusively, a hospital contemplating corrective action for a practitioner must provide that person with notice that states the following:

- That a professional review action has been proposed
- The reasons for the proposed action
- The time limit (not less than 30 days) within which the physician must request a hearing
- A summary of the practitioner's rights in the hearing process

If a hearing is requested, the practitioner must be given timely notice of its place, time, and date, along with a list of witnesses expected to testify. The hearing must be conducted before either a mutually acceptable arbitrator, a hearing officer appointed by the hospital who is not in direct economic competition with the practitioner, or a panel of individuals appointed by the hospital who are not in direct economic competition with the practitioner involved.

At the hearing, the physician has the right to be represented by a lawyer or other person of the physician's choosing, to have a record made of the proceedings, to call and cross-examine witnesses, to present evidence determined to be relevant, and to submit a written statement at the close of the hearing. After the hearing, the practitioner has the right to receive a written recommendation of the arbitrator, officer, or panel, including a statement of the basis for the recommendation, and to receive a written decision from the hospital, including a written statement of the basis for the decision.

If the hospital's decision is based on a *reasonable belief* that the action was warranted by the facts after a reasonable effort has been made to obtain the facts and if the *notice and hearing procedures* described in the act are followed, the immunity promised by the act will be invoked. The trouble with the act is that the question of whether the hospital (and other defendants) has met these conditions for immunity is one that can result in months of pretrial discovery and days or weeks of trial. If Congress's objective in passing the law was to remove the spectre of litigation, it missed the mark by a mile.

On the other hand, the Health Care Quality Improvement Act does provide a level of welcome protection in the federal antitrust arena. Before the act was passed, hospitals, doctors, and possibly board members could, if the conditions were right, find themselves facing the treble damages of federal civil antitrust suits as a result of good-faith credentialing decisions that had an anticompetitive effect. Under the act, this danger is gone as long as credentialing decisions are based on a reasonable belief that they promote high-quality health care, and aggrieved practitioners have a fair opportunity to present their cases.

In any event, the Health Care Quality Improvement Act is the only statutory protection available to limit the liability of directors in federal law cases. But in the instance of medical staff credentialing disputes under state law, which constitute the numerically greatest danger to directors, the act requires too much and gives too little. Protection such as that afforded under the Illinois law described earlier is far broader and far less demanding.

Board Actions to Strengthen Immunity

Despite their preconditions and limitations, immunity laws can provide a first line of defense against the risk of director liability. To get the most out of these protective devices, there are some basic things that hospital directors should do.

Know the Law, How It Works, and What It Requires

With the exception of the Health Care Quality Improvement Act, the laws that limit director liability are enacted at the state level, and the description provided here is, of necessity, too broad to provide more than a general idea of what might be encompassed by the law of any given state. But directors should have this information, and boards should instruct their hospital administrators to get it for them as it relates to their corporations and their states. Each director should be provided with a clear and understandable description of any immunity laws that apply to the hospital's board and of what these laws require in order to be activated.

Take Action to Benefit from the Law

Although many laws providing director immunity are self-executing, there may be instances in which some further action on the part of the board is needed in order to meet conditions necessary for the protection or to prevent its loss. These steps should be identified for the board. Where there are trade-offs—such as the need to forfeit some right or to follow burdensome procedures—in order to gain immunity, the advisability of making them should be considered and discussed by the board. The board should then take the action needed to gain or prevent the loss of immunity to the extent it deems such action to be advisable.

Promote the Passage of State Laws

Not all states have passed laws like those described here to protect hospital directors, and often the laws that states have passed are not as helpful as they could be. Where this is so, state and regional hospital associations should be urged to sponsor and promote new or amended protective state enabling legislation, and hospital directors should lend their support to these association efforts.

As we pointed out at the beginning of this section, although statutes limiting director liability may not be a panacea, some protection is better than none at all. Opponents of these laws brand them as a means of letting corporate directors off the hook and say that these laws simply serve to reduce the risk to director and officer liability insurance companies. Hospital directors, however, may view these laws in a different light, and by pushing for and supporting hospital association efforts to gain greater legal protection, directors can help reduce the personal risk of serving the community through hospital board involvement.

Indemnity

Indemnity is the second "eye" of director protection. It comes into play when all else has failed, and a claim naming the board or certain directors is made and losses are incurred. Under the concept of director indemnity, the corporation pays the losses an individual suffers as a result of serving as a director or makes restitution or reimbursement for amounts paid by the individual.

Director indemnification has not always been a feature of the corporate landscape. In an earlier era lawsuits against directors occurred so infrequently that few people felt a need for this protection. Suits alleging a breach of the duty of care were virtual losers due to the protection afforded by the business judgment rule. Suits based on breaches of the duties of loyalty and obedience were the kinds that most frequently touched directors, but directors involved as defendants in these kinds of suits were not always thought by their corporations to be deserving of protection. Thus, prior to the current era, few states even bothered to place on their books enabling legislation allowing corporations to indemnify directors.

Such enabling statutes are considered a necessary prerequisite for director indemnification. If a board authorized indemnification of directors without specific statutory permission, it might be argued that the board was breaching its fiduciary duty of loyalty to the corporation by using corporate resources for the benefit of directors.

Over the past 20 years, this situation has undergone dramatic change, however. Today, the corporation laws of virtually every state *authorize* corporations to indemnify corporate directors and officers for a broad range of expenses and damages suffered as a result of board service.

It is important to note, however, that the scope of corporate indemnification permitted by statute varies from state to state and can be different for the different types of corporations. Some kinds of losses—fines for criminal conduct, for example, and expenses for the unsuccessful defense of criminal charges—are frequently outside the range of protection permitted by the state statutes.

Corporate Bylaws to Grant Indemnification

It is also important to note that the state statutes generally *authorize* rather than *require* corporations to indemnify directors when liability claims arise. This distinction is of utmost importance for directors. The fact that a corporation is authorized to indemnify directors does not mean that it will choose to do so in every case. For this reason, prudent boards take care to ensure that the bylaws or charter of the corporation contain provisions requiring the corporation to indemnify directors to the limits permitted by state law whenever director liability arises.

Some will argue that this sort of blanket assurance of indemnification deprives a board of making case-by-case determinations of when restitution should be made and that undeserving directors may, therefore, end up receiving protection when the board would prefer to deny it. This argument may sound good, but individual directors—especially those serving in a voluntary capacity—may see the situation a little differently. They may ask, "For what reason should a director who has no personal stake in a corporation ever place personal assets at risk by leaving the decision of whether indemnification should be made to the discretion or whim of some future board?" To the degree that directors can influence or control the bylaws, they should not leave this protection to chance.

If permitted by state law, the corporate bylaws should also specify that the legal defense costs incurred by directors will be paid directly by the corporation and that any expenses paid by directors will be reimbursed on an interim basis following request by the director. Without such a bylaw requirement in place, a director may be denied expense reimbursement by the corporation until the legal matter is concluded—often years after it commences. In this situation directors can find themselves confronting ruinous legal defense expenses that can wipe out personal savings. Such expenses can also render it impossible for the director to mount a winning legal defense, an element sometimes required under state law in order for indemnification to be made.

At this point many directors may be thinking, "Hey, my board of directors would never leave me in this kind of lurch. Why should I be concerned about what our bylaws say about required indemnification?" The answer is based on a core reality of director liability: Most successful suits against directors are brought by, or in the name of, the corporation. These suits are frequently brought after there has been a major change in the composition of the board of directors. Thus, the corporation the sued director looks to for indemnification is likely to be the plaintiff in the suit, and the new board of directors of the corporation is likely to be extremely antagonistic. Under these circumstances, "nice" just doesn't happen. If a director wants comfort that the protection of indemnification will be granted in these instances, the actions described above are essential.

Board Action to Ensure Protection

All of this discussion about what should be contained in corporate bylaws raises two interesting questions for boards: What level of indemnification is permitted under the state law governing the corporation? What do the bylaws of the hospital corporation currently say about indemnification? Answers to both of these questions require some unpleasant work.

The statutory and bylaw language typically used to describe the nature of the indemnification that will be made to directors appears to have been drafted first by a Groucho Marx parody of a lawyer and then cloned and passed along to infest the statutes of the various states and the bylaws of corporations throughout America. The language tends to be dreadfully boring and difficult to comprehend. Unfortunately, it has to be read by somebody, and the following is an action plan that boards should consider:

- As a starting point, a hospital board should instruct its administrator to have prepared for the board's review a legal interpretation of the kind of indemnification permitted by the state corporation law under which the hospital corporation is organized.
- The board should also require a legal interpretation of the indemnification provisions found in the corporation's own bylaws.
- These interpretations should be accompanied by an analysis pointing out for the board those things that can be done to broaden and strengthen the corporation's director indemnification program.
- The interpretations and analysis should be subjected to careful consideration and discussion by the board, ideally through assignment to a standing or ad hoc board committee. This committee should develop recommendations for changes in the bylaws of the corporation for consideration by the full board, and a plan for effecting changes in the corporate documents should also be developed and implemented.

Of course, winning effective changes in corporate indemnification provisions is not always easy. Some boards may not agree that the maximum indemnification protection possible should be granted automatically. Bylaw changes may require approval from corporate members, which is not always easy to obtain. Or there may be other obstacles to change.

Where there is an unwillingness to grant or an impossibility of obtaining an adequate level of indemnification protection, however, individual hospital directors are free to make their own decisions on whether to continue serving on the board. Many directors will probably accept the risk involved and remain in service. What is important, however, is that directors make these decisions on an educated basis, and an action plan like the one set out above will make this possible.

Shortcomings of Indemnification

Indemnification can protect directors against certain risks that director and officer liability insurance policies may not cover. However, it cannot provide blanket financial protection to directors in all cases.

For one thing, a promise or commitment to indemnify is only as good as the financial capabilities of the party who has the obligation. If a hospital corporation falls on hard times, it may simply lack the financial wherewithal to make good on its indemnification commitment. For another, state statutes, which authorize corporate indemnification in the first place, may exclude certain kinds of conduct from indemnification coverage. In private foundations and public corporations, state law may consider indemnification to constitute prohibited self-dealing. Indemnification for settlements and judgments in derivative suits may also be prohibited.

Thus, as important as indemnification is for protecting hospital directors against personal liability, it leaves gaps in its coverage. Some of these gaps can be filled by director and officer liability insurance coverage.

Insurance

Director and officer (D&O) liability insurance coverage is the third "eye" of director protection. This coverage can provide financial backup for the indemnification pledges made by hospital corporations to their directors and can fill some of the gaps left in a hospital corporation's board indemnification program. However, D&O coverage on its own does not provide complete protection to directors for all of the potential liability to which they are exposed.

Prior to the liability insurance crisis of the mid-1980s, D&O coverage was widely available at a reasonable cost, and the scope of coverage was fairly broad and inclusive. Liability limits were high, and extended coverage could be obtained to cover many of the events excluded under standard policies. When the insurance crisis hit, availability dried up, premiums jumped dramatically, the scope of coverage was reduced, and the form of insurance was changed from *occurrence* to *claims made* in most cases. (Claims-made coverage only provides protection against claims made during the policy period during which the insurance is in effect.) With the passing of the crisis, availability opened up and prices came down, but the coverage limitations generally stayed in place, and the claims-made form remained the insurance coverage most widely offered.

Hospital directors tend to leave insurance matters to the chief financial officer or hospital risk manager, but there are some important things they should know and concern themselves with.

Limitations on Coverage

D&O insurance policies contain provisions describing the parties and the general events covered by the insurance contract. They also list specific events and claims that are excluded from coverage unless extended coverage is purchased.

In chapter 2, we pointed out that many of the claims typically excluded from standard D&O insurance policies are those that pose the greatest risk for hospital directors. These may include:

- Discrimination in employment
- Medical staff credentialing
- Environmental violations
- Antitrust violations

Thus, unless extended coverage can be obtained, D&O coverage for directors will fail to provide the fullest possible protection. Coverage of some events, such as illegal activities by directors, may never be available, either because such coverage is prohibited by state law or because insurance companies refuse to insure losses that are considered under the control of individual directors.

Claims-Made Coverage

Under the claims-made coverage form of insurance, a director has no assurance that D&O coverage will be in place at some future date when a claim is actually made. Say, for example, that a controversial board action is taken in 1990. The board has made sure that the corporation obtained D&O coverage that would protect against liability that might arise from the decision. The coverage is written in the claims-made form, the only insurance form available.

No claim is made in the 1990 policy year, but the following year there is a major turnover in board composition, and the new board either drops

D&O coverage or fails to purchase extended coverage that would continue liability protection for the controversial decision. A suit is then filed during the new policy year naming the former directors. They are out of luck. The claims-made policy in effect in 1990 is no longer valid, and the new claims-made policy excludes the event in question from coverage. The new board could have continued the full coverage in effect under the new insurance contract, or it could have purchased "tail" coverage to extend the protection offered in 1990 into the future, but it did neither.

Claims-Notice Provisions

Insurance policies set forth the time and manner in which directors protected under D&O coverage must notify the insurance carrier of claims filed against them. Failure to abide by these notice provisions can result in a denial of coverage even if the event giving rise to the claim is supposed to be protected under the policy.

What the Board Should Do about Insurance Coverage

There is no reason or excuse for hospital boards to leave their protection from risk to chance. This is an area where boards can and should help themselves reduce their exposure to personal financial loss. Most of the activities listed here should be undertaken at least annually.

Learn and Understand the Scope of D&O Insurance

As in the case of state and federal immunity laws and indemnification matters, the board should require the hospital administrator to obtain and provide an understandable description of the coverage afforded under the D&O insurance program provided by the corporation. Indeed, this description should be tied in with a description of the protection provided under the hospital's director indemnification plan, so that directors can fully understand and appreciate any voids existing in the combined protection. Anything less leaves the directors playing a potentially risky game with less than a full deck.

Learn the Insurance Notice Requirements

A description of the D&O insurance policy should include the rules and information required to file notice of a liability claim with the insurance company. Directors should never rely on someone else to file required notices with the insurance carrier on their behalf.

Provide for Continuity of Coverage

Boards should also require that legal counsel for the corporation devise ways to ensure that full D&O insurance protection is continued into the future, so that directors aren't left with diminished D&O insurance protection after they leave the board. Special bylaw or charter provisions or individual contracts between directors and the hospital corporation may provide a means for ensuring this continuity of coverage.

Study and Undertake Corrective Action

Finally, the board, through a standing or ad hoc committee, should study and evaluate the profile of protections and voids resulting from the combination of indemnification and insurance provisions. The purpose of this process is to determine shortcomings and develop corrective action that can be implemented by the full board. If the board lacks the expertise, it should seek the assistance of the hospital's lawyers and insurance consultants.

The Bottom Line for Limiting Risk

It would be irresponsible to play down the risk of direct personal liability for hospital directors in today's environment, and yet the preceding materials should provide comfort. Directors who take their jobs seriously and carry out their duties with loyalty and care have only a limited exposure to risk.

If the states in which their hospitals are incorporated have had the good sense to provide meaningful immunity to corporate directors, the risk is further reduced. The remaining exposure can be covered through effective indemnification and insurance strategies that boards themselves can foster and implement.

Beyond maximizing the protection offered by the "three eyes," however, there are a number of liability prevention strategies that boards can also employ. The areas of hospital director liability exposure that pose the greatest dollar risk are the ones that deserve the greatest attention. Those areas and related strategies are dealt with in the next three chapters of this book.

☐ References

1. Smith v. Van Gorkom, 488 A.2d 858.
2. Shaw, B. Statutory limits on director liability. *Business Horizons* 32:43–50, July–Aug. 1989.
3. Illinois Revised Statutes, ch. 32, paragraph 108.70(a).
4. Illinois Revised Statutes, ch. 32, paragraph 108.70(d).
5. Illinois Revised Statutes, ch. 111½, paragraph 151.2.
6. Patrick v. Burget, 486 U.S. 94, 108 S. Ct. 1658 (1988).

Chapter 5

Medical Staff Credentialing

Chapter 2 talked about the good news and the bad news of hospital director liability. Chapter 3 described the legal duties directors are expected to meet. Chapter 4 told about three "eyes" that can limit the personal liability to which hospital directors might otherwise be exposed. In the next three chapters we look at some specific things that hospital directors should do to keep the liability "wolf" away from their door. We will begin with medical staff credentialing.

Medical Staff Credentialing

Medical staff credentialing is one of the hospital board's most important jobs. It is also one of the jobs that boards know least about and do least well. Yet directors are smack in the middle of the credentialing process. They have authority to control the medical staff bylaws, they pass on applications for appointment and reappointment, and they play an active role when corrective actions are taken concerning a practitioner on the medical staff.

Considering all of this and the dire financial and professional consequences of adverse credentialing decisions on medical practitioners, it is hardly surprising that directors are sued occasionally by doctors made unhappy by medical staff credentialing actions. In these instances hospital directors are like sitting ducks.

But perhaps the subject of this book causes us to view this topic of medical staff credentialing from the wrong perspective. Although director liability is a legitimate concern, the real reason that hospital boards must pay closer attention to medical staff credentialing is that effective credentialing is the keystone of high-quality hospital care. In theory, directors could find themselves liable to the hospital corporation if they failed to exercise their duty of care in the credentialing arena. Theory aside, however, hospitals will frequently find themselves in trouble when directors fail in their credentialing chores.

What Is Medical Staff Credentialing?

American health care has invented a vocabulary of its own largely because many of the things that occur in the health care environment have no readily identifiable counterparts elsewhere in our society. Credentialing is a perfect example of this phenomenon. In most dictionaries the word *credential* is not a verb, and the word *credentialing* doesn't exist. Health care has fabricated these words to describe a complex process that is as unique to health care as *vetting* is to government security organizations.

Hospital medical staff credentialing is really more than a procedure. *It is a combination of rules, forms, processes, documentation, and reports aimed at assessing the overall professionalism of practitioners allowed to care for patients in a hospital setting. It is an ongoing activity encompassing appointment and reappointment to the medical staff, continual monitoring and evaluation, corrective or disciplinary action when a practitioner's conduct falls short of an acceptable level of professionalism, and internal review mechanisms to ensure fairness.*

This is pretty heady stuff, and it is little wonder that most hospital directors—even those with years of service—are befuddled when they approach the credentialing arena. They are usually more than happy to "delegate" credentialing to the medical staff and administration and, instead, busy themselves with other important hospital business that falls more comfortably into their realm of knowledge and experience.

What boards may fail to understand is that the hospital medical staff and administration are only marginally better equipped to handle credentialing than is the board. Within the medical staff, *credentialing* is generally thought of as the peer review acts of reviewing and evaluating. This work is typically performed by doctors who volunteer for a few years through service on one or another of the medical staff committees—departmental, credentialing, or executive.

What these doctors do best is practice medicine. Only seldom do they ever receive formal training in medical staff credentialing. Their education in this regard is more often the occasional, hands-on experience gained in the committee, which means that what they learn reflects what has gone on in the institution in the past. Boards tend to view the medical staff as expert and knowledgeable about credentialing, but they're usually wrong.

Administration may be slightly more knowledgeable than the medical staff regarding credentialing, but its role generally clerical—that of gathering information, passing paper, and keeping records. These clerical functions are typically assigned to secretarial personnel. This is not to say that they are performed poorly. Secretaries involved in medical staff credentialing are often the strongest spoke in the credentialing wheel—smart, motivated, hardworking, and frustrated—frustrated because they, too, receive no formal training and lack the authority to improve their (or anybody else's) piece of the credentialing whole.

In hospitals with salaried medical directors or other administrative personnel whose specific duties include credentialing, things may be somewhat better than portrayed here. Yet, even in the most advanced institutions, progress is only now being made in viewing credentialing in its broadest context:

- To integrate the results of hospital quality assurance activities into credentialing for purposes of reappointment or positive corrective action programs
- To ensure that credentialing rules provide for effective credentialing, meet legal requirements, and are followed within the institution
- To ensure that forms used in credentialing—applications, verifications, reference checks, checklists, and others—do the job they're intended to do
- To ensure that the documentation of credentialing complies with the institution's credentialing rules and results in a comprehensive record of credentialing actions
- To ensure that the processes used in credentialing meet internal and external rules, integrate all relevant information, and result in fair and effective credentialing decisions
- To ensure that medical staff members with problems in professional performance are identified early and are provided with positive assistance aimed at correcting the problem and maintaining medical staff membership when possible

The Traditional Board Role in Credentialing

Boards traditionally have played a very limited role in medical staff credentialing. Were this otherwise, the mystery surrounding the board's role in credentialing today would probably not exist. After all, hospital finance is complex and confusing to outsiders, but hospital directors have always tackled this subject and have had little difficulty knowing and understanding how it fits into the board's activities.

But in modern hospital history, medical staff credentialing commonly has been viewed as a medical staff activity for which the board was legally but not functionally responsible. Indeed, this division of responsibilities has long been recognized and institutionalized by the Joint Commission on Accreditation of Healthcare Organizations and by the hospital licensing regulations of many states.

In the parlance of the day, medical staff credentialing is delegated to the medical staff, and the role of the board is to act upon the recommendations of the medical staff. The board's authority is recognized as supreme, but its function, in practice, is to rubber-stamp that which comes before it. When so much is at stake, one might ask whether this is the practice of the reasonably prudent. Commentators in the field are calling this practice into question with increasing frequency, and hospital directors, among others, increasingly show themselves to be concerned with this role. But when they ask, "What are we supposed to do?" the answers are not always very helpful or clear.

Comparing the Credentialing Role with Other Roles

Before going on to consider what hospital directors ought to be doing to play an appropriately active role in medical staff credentialing, let's take time out for an exercise that may put the subject in a helpful perspective. Experienced hospital directors have their own views of which board activities are the most important, and these views can be determined by the fairly simple questionnaire in figure 5-1. The ratings would vary from director to director and from hospital to hospital, but, hypothetically, they might be portrayed as in figure 5-2.

Figure 5-1. Sample Questionnaire to Determine Board Views on the Importance of Various Activities

What's Important?
Rate each of the following possible board functions by indicating whether you think it is very important (10), moderately important (5), of minor importance (1), or something in between.

Possible Board Function	Minor	Moderate	Very
Safeguarding the hospital's financial resources	1 2 3	4 5 6 7	8 9 10
Mission and planning	1 2 3	4 5 6 7	8 9 10
Operations/new program feasibility review	1 2 3	4 5 6 7	8 9 10
Ensuring high-quality medical staff	1 2 3	4 5 6 7	8 9 10
Hospital quality assurance	1 2 3	4 5 6 7	8 9 10
CEO selection and evaluation	1 2 3	4 5 6 7	8 9 10
Board management and education	1 2 3	4 5 6 7	8 9 10
Medical staff recruitment and relations	1 2 3	4 5 6 7	8 9 10
Fund-raising and community relations	1 2 3	4 5 6 7	8 9 10
Buildings and grounds, new construction	1 2 3	4 5 6 7	8 9 10
Hospital personnel matters (other than financial)	1 2 3	4 5 6 7	8 9 10

Medical Staff Credentialing

Figure 5-2. Sample Bar Graph Rating the Importance of Board Functions

Board Function	Minor	Moderate	Very
	1 2 3	4 5 6 7 8	9 10
Safeguarding the hospital's financial resources	■■■■■■■■■■■■■■■■■■■■■■■■■■■■		
Mission and planning	■■■■■■■■■■■■■■■■■■■■■■		
Operations/new program feasibility review	■■■■■■■■■■■		
Ensuring high-quality medical staff	■■■■■■■■■■■■■■■■■■■■■■■■■■■		
Hospital quality assurance	■■■■■■■■■■■■■■■■■■■■■■■■■■		
CEO selection and evaluation	■■■■■■■■■■■■■■■■■■■■■■■■■■■		
Board management and education	■■■■■■■■■■■■		
Medical staff recruitment and relations	■■■■■■■■■■		
Fund-raising and community relations	■■■■■■		
Buildings and grounds, new construction	■■■■■■		
Hospital personnel matters (other than financial)	■■■■■■■■■■■		

Directors also know roughly how much time the board and its committees devote to the various governance functions, and the percentage of the board's time—its most important resource—spent on each function can likewise be determined through a questionnaire. Information concerning standing committees devoted to specific governance functions and whether hospital staff management specialists are assigned to the functions administratively can also be determined.

The graph resulting from such a series of questions provides an interesting and valuable illustration of how the board's and the hospital's resources are deployed to meet the functions the board considers most important. The graph of a hypothetical, typical hospital might look something like figure 5-3.

Figure 5-3. Sample Bar Graph Comparing the Importance Ratings in Figure 5-2 with Time Spent on Board Functions

Scales:	■■■■■■■■■■ Importance ■■■■■■■■■■
	Minor　　　　　　　Moderate　　　　　　Very
	1　2　3　4　5　6　7　8　9　10
	★★★★★★★★ Percentage of Board Time ★★★★★★★★
	0　　　　10　　　　20　　　　30　　　　40

Board Function	
Safeguarding the hospital's financial resources[1,2]	■■■■■■■■■■■■■■■■■■■■■■■■■■■■■■■■■ ★★★★★★★★★★★★★★★★★★★★★★★★★★★★★★★★★
Mission and planning[1]	■■■■■■■■■■■■■■■■■■■■ ★★★★★★★★★★★★
Operations/new program feasibility review[2]	■■■■■■■■■■■■■ ★★★★★★★★★★★★
Ensuring high-quality medical staff	■■■■■■■■■■■■■■■■■■■■■■■■■■■■■ ★★
Hospital quality assurance[1,2]	■■■■■■■■■■■■■■■■■■■■■■■■■■■ ★★★★
CEO selection and evaluation	■■■■■■■■■■■■■■■■■■■■■■■■■■■ ★★
Board management and education	■■■■■■■■■■■■■■ ★★★★★
Medical staff recruitment and relations	■■■■■■■■■■ ★★★★★
Fund-raising and community relations[1,2]	■■■■■■■ ★★★★★
Buildings and grounds, new construction[1,2]	■■■■■■■ ★★★★
Hospital personnel matters (other than financial)[1,2]	■■■■■■■■■■■ ★★★

[1]A specialized board committee has been assigned to the function.
[2]A dedicated administrative manager has been assigned to the function.

To be sure, these time percentages (and other resource allocations) will vary from place to place and from time to time. A board that is replacing its chief executive officer will spend a great deal of time on the search and will probably create an ad hoc committee to oversee the process. An institution with labor unions will devote a good deal of board time and attention to personnel matters, and the board of a hospital engaged in a major building program will focus increased time resources on fund-raising and project review. And a hospital with medical staff quality problems will be forced to spend great quantities of time dealing with corrective action matters.

In the main, however, the hypothetical graph in figure 5-3 reflects the norm. Boards devote their greatest attention to finance. Resources devoted to planning and operations generally correspond to the importance boards place on their involvement in these matters. Due to external pressures, boards are now spending greater time and other resources on institutional quality assurance matters. But when it comes to ensuring a high-quality medical staff—the object of medical staff credentialing—hospital directors typically and traditionally pay only scant attention, despite their awareness and understanding of the importance of their involvement.

What the Board Should Do about Credentialing

Each reader undoubtedly will make a personal evaluation of the validity of this graphic portrayal. If there is one point on which most will agree, however, it is that hospital boards make their greatest efforts and have their greatest successes in the area of finance. This is the function in which hospital boards most often shine. Let's take a closer look at what boards do or cause to be done in finance and see whether any lessons can be learned for application in the area of medical staff credentialing.

The *first lesson* is that the success of hospital boards in the area of finance has little to do with direct involvement in financial management. Boards don't mess around with the financial books and records of the hospital. They don't send and collect bills or pay the bills of vendors.

What boards do is to make sure that the hospital corporation has an experienced and competent chief financial officer to organize and manage the financial function. They provide this person with the personnel, equipment, and consulting and other resources necessary to operate a modern and effective finance department. This is the *second lesson*. Find a board that excels at finance and you will likely find a first-rate hospital finance department. If the board failed to do these things, however, there is no way the directors could make up for the chaos that would result.

This is not to say, however, that hospital boards are merely satisfied with an excellent finance staff. Directors educate themselves to know and understand the most important things about hospital finance. They learn about Medicare, Medicaid, and insurance reimbursement as well as standards for accounts receivable, length of stay, depreciation, cash flow, investment strategies, capital debt, monitors and ratios, and hundreds of other things necessary to understand what is going on in the hospital's financial operations. This is *lesson three*. Without understanding hospital finance, the board would be hard-pressed to do the things in lessons four and five below.

Boards set goals for the hospital's financial performance through the budgeting process. They don't do this alone, but in conjunction with the hospital's operating and financial managers, based on what appears realistic and achievable. But by setting these goals they create a measurement against which performance can be evaluated, the *fourth lesson* for elaboration later in this chapter.

Fifth, boards *monitor* financial performance with great scrutiny on a regular, continuing basis. They require detailed financial *reports,* and they spend a great deal of time analyzing and discussing these reports with hospital management and providing directives for management action—further goals and further monitoring. Problems are detected early, and action is taken early to resolve them.

These tasks of education, goal setting, and monitoring take lots of time, and boards devoté this time because the job of finance is so important to the success of the corporation. They make finance a board priority. This prioritizing and devotion of director time is the *sixth lesson* to be gained.

The time commitment and specialized knowledge required to perform complex responsibilities well can be overly burdensome to the board as a whole. Thus, hospital boards designate a separate standing committee made up of members who bring knowledge of finance to the table or who can learn and who can devote the time necessary to carry out the boards' role effectively. In most instances, it would be impossible for the full board to perform the work of the finance committee as well as the other work of the board during the course of regular meetings. The use of a specialized committee is the *seventh lesson* to be gained from the involvement of hospital boards in finance.

Finally, once a year, at substantial expense, the board brings in an outside auditor to review the hospital's financial records and practices to ensure that they meet standards of accuracy and acceptability. The auditor also provides a management report containing recommendations to correct shortcomings uncovered in the organization's financial management.

When operational problems requiring specialized expertise or time commitments beyond the capabilities of financial administrators arise, hospital boards also authorize the use of outside help. The use of auditors and other independent experts to assist the board in its monitoring role is the *eighth lesson* to be learned from the area of finance.

Reviewing these eight lessons against board practices in the area of medical staff credentialing should make clear the reasons for the disparity in board performance between these two critical functions. It will also provide direction for necessary changes that hospital boards should consider.

Lesson One. Boards don't do the work of administrators or the medical staff.

To carry out the board's function in medical staff credentialing, it is neither necessary nor desirable for boards to perform administrative or peer review operations. Aside from the education that can be gained by sitting in on medical staff credentialing deliberations or sifting through the files and forms of practitioners undergoing review, there is little reason for directors to play any greater role in medical staff credentialing than they play in the hospital's financial operation. This is not the board's role, and in the long run directors who cross the line into operations and peer review are more of a detriment than a help.

An exception may arise when credentialing decisions are appealed to the board. For better or worse, tradition often places directors in the role of final arbitrators in these appeals. Obviously, if the hospital's credentialing rules place directors in this role, it is one they must play and play well. Otherwise, boards should steer clear of the nitty-gritty work of credentialing.

Lesson Two. Boards provide specialized personnel and resources.

There is no substitute for knowledgeable administrative staff specialists and physicians equipped with the resources necessary to do their jobs. Alas, few are the hospitals where such staff is provided for medical staff credentialing and, as pointed out earlier, doctors are seldom trained in peer review.

Disparaging the efforts of the doctors and the secretaries who work hard and selflessly in medical staff credentialing is the last thing this author would want to do. But the simple fact is that, with few exceptions, dumping the bulk of the chore of medical staff credentialing off onto untrained physician volunteers and medical staff or administrative secretaries doesn't cut it in today's world.

Perhaps the tradition surrounding medical staff credentialing and the institutionalization of practices brought about by the Joint Commission and state regulations foreclose dramatic changes in the practice of "delegation." At the very least, however, hospital directors can take steps to ensure that the "delegates" are provided with the knowledge necessary to perform their functions with skill and proficiency.

Hospitals with adequate resources can also engage knowledgeable medical staff directors to run the credentialing system or engage outside organizations to take over part of the credentialing burden. This does not mean that the review and evaluation—the peer review function—performed by the medical staff should be changed. With training, doctors are best equipped to perform this task. It does mean, however, that the rest of credentialing—the rules, forms, processes, documentation, and reports that form the nonevaluative part of credentialing operations—should be handled by people who know what they're doing. Otherwise, how can the board possibly be confident that the job is being done right?

Lesson Three. Boards educate themselves.

Few people who join hospital boards already know and understand medical staff credentialing. The rules, forms, processes, documentation, and reports surrounding credentialing just aren't found outside the hospital environment, and the whole system is so specialized that it probably lies outside the normal intuitive range of most people, no matter what their background. Boards can hardly play a proper role on the basis of this ignorance, and a systematic program of education is essential, just as it is in hospital finance.

The process does not occur overnight, and it takes more than just hands-on experience. The hospital must underwrite and directors must participate in an ongoing educational process that eventually covers all aspects of the medical staff credentialing system. This range includes federal, state, and accreditation rules; institutional rules, processes, and documentation dealing with appointments, reappointments, and corrective action; problems; and problem solving. Books, articles, retreats, guest speakers, and seminars are all means that can be used to provide this education, with one caution: Finding good materials and programs on credentialing is still a challenge.

Lesson Four. Boards set goals.

Nobody said this would be easy! And setting goals in medical staff credentialing may not be as commonplace as it is in finance, where performance goals are the name of the game. Nonetheless, the setting of meaningful goals brings credentialing right to the center of the board's proper playing field, and it is an essential line in the board's role.

A short example: Under the Health Care Quality Improvement Act, hospitals are required to submit certain kinds of information to, and request certain kinds of medical staff credentialing information from, a federal data bank. The hospital board knows this, the administrator knows this, and the medical staff credentialing committee knows this, but nobody has thought about who should be responsible for keeping up and complying with the federal requirements. The board suggests that the administrator should sort this question out with the medical staff and report on the outcome at the next meeting. It is so done and reported. A knowledgeable board sets a goal, and there is performance monitoring and reporting — one small step on the road to perfection (or at least problem avoidance).

But this example may serve to understate the ambition here. In many institutions medical staff credentialing has serious problems that must be addressed. Internal rules fall short of external requirements, processes don't work, forms fail to elicit proper information, credentialing personnel are ill-prepared, quality assurance results are not considered in reappointment assessments, and documentation is inadequate. Every one of these problems translates into a goal, and the identification of the credentialing system's problems may be the most significant initial goal of all.

As hospital boards come to play their proper role in medical staff credentialing, they must realize that in many cases they are entering virgin territory. Like pioneers, they must fell the trees and clear the rocks before they can plow the soil and grow prize crops. Thus, the goals they first set may, of necessity, be rudimentary. As their involvement matures and their knowledge increases, the goals will turn to fine-tuning.

One thing that causes boards difficulty in setting goals in this area is the lack of a mission or purpose statement covering medical staff credentialing. Look around your hospital. The likelihood is that nobody has ever defined and set down what medical staff credentialing should accomplish. If nobody knows where they want to go, it's difficult to set goals that will take them anywhere. Some points that may be used in a board's mission or purpose statement for medical staff credentialing system are these:

- The medical staff credentialing system should ensure that only persons who are appropriately licensed and clinically competent, who demonstrate their ability to work constructively with all co-workers, who treat their patients in a professionally efficient manner, and who are physically and mentally capable of providing continuous care for patients in the hospital are permitted to join and remain on the medical staff.
- Clinical privileges of members of the medical staff must reflect their known, current levels of competence.
- The rules and processes used in medical staff credentialing must meet all external requirements.
- All aspects of medical staff credentialing decisions and actions must be fully and clearly documented, and all documentation concerning medical staff members and applicants for membership must be maintained in the practitioner's file.
- The rules and processes used in the medical staff credentialing decisions and actions concerning practitioners must be fair and impartial.
- The medical staff credentialing system must be effective at early identification of practitioners with problems that affect their professionalism so that corrective assistance can be provided when it is appropriate.
- The medical staff credentialing system should be designed to minimize the demands on medical staff members who volunteer their time for peer review.
- The medical staff credentialing system should uncover and provide for the expeditious review and handling of serious problems.
- The medical staff credentialing system and the reports given to the board of directors should lend themselves to effectiveness monitoring by the board.

The establishment of a medical staff credentialing mission or purpose statement for many boards falls into the "tree-clearing" goal category mentioned earlier. It's the kind of rudimentary goal that must be established before other, more operational goals can be contemplated. A second tree-clearing goal is to identify the strengths and weaknesses of the credentialing system currently in place in the hospital. This second goal will be discussed in greater detail in lesson eight.

Lesson Five. The board monitors whether goals are being reached.

Everybody knows that a key role of the board in medical staff credentialing is that of monitoring. The question is, monitoring what? When there are no goals, the tendency of boards is to monitor everything or nothing. It is not uncommon for hospital boards to devote the final 5 or 10 minutes of their meetings to pass on medical staff recommendations. Not much monitoring going on there.

Whether they attempt to monitor everything or nothing, however, directors waste their time and energy and come away frustrated and confused. This is certainly not the way the boards operate in the area of finance. Indeed, as with finance, effective monitoring in medical staff credentialing is the corollary of goal setting: checking performance to ensure that goals and standards have been met and taking corrective action when they haven't been.

The board's principal tool for monitoring performance in this area is reports from the people who are responsible for doing the tasks required to make the hospital's medical staff credentialing system work. Unfortunately, a full discussion of the subjects that should be covered by these reports and the kind of information these reports should contain is beyond the modest scope of this book.

Reporting in an effective medical staff credentialing system, however, should be every bit as comprehensive in its own way as the reporting used in the area of finance. Especially important are the reports provided to the board in connection with board actions covering appointments to the medical staff, appointment denials, reappointments, leaves of absence, clinical privileges, and corrective action. In each case, the report is intended to support board action that could have a lasting effect on the practitioner involved and on the hospital. Each director's legal duty of care requires that these reports provide the board with adequate information upon which to make a reasonably informed judgment. As goals and objectives are established for the medical staff credentialing system, other report mechanisms should provide the board with information upon which to monitor progress and to gauge the overall activity and performance of the system.

Lesson Six. Boards spend time on important activities.

The graphic portrayal shown earlier in this chapter tells the story: Boards generally spend large amounts of time on finance and minuscule amounts of time on medical staff credentialing. Obviously, the devotion of large amounts of time in itself is not enough to guarantee positive results. But without the allocation of adequate time and the prioritizing this time reflects, it is impossible to learn and master the job.

Lesson Seven. Boards use a specialized committee.

Boards use committees to do their difficult and time-consuming work. Besides freeing the rest of the board so that valuable time can be devoted to broader policy issues, the committee structure lends itself to the development of the specialized expertise and knowledge necessary to do a particular job well. Just as most hospital boards use committees for their other big jobs such as finance, they should use committees of board members for medical staff credentialing.

Most boards don't do this, and the thought of another demanding committee assignment is not pleasant to most directors. But consider the alternatives: Without the use of a specialized committee, either the board as a whole must devote more time to medical staff credentialing, or the job just won't get done.

Lesson Eight. Boards make use of independent review.

Given the shortfall in board involvement and knowledge in medical staff credentialing, this may be the most important lesson of all. In the area of finance, boards authorize the use of outside auditors and experts to verify and validate financial systems and data and to provide guidance in problem solving and systems development. Boards don't try to do this work themselves, and they don't rely solely on administrative staff either. This approach can be very helpful—maybe essential—in medical staff credentialing.

An independent audit or review of a hospital's medical staff credentialing system, for example, can provide the board, administration, and medical staff with an objective, top-to-bottom review and analysis of the system that points out problems and sets forth an action plan for improvement. This result helps the board to work with the administration and the medical staff to set performance goals as described in lesson four. The board can then monitor performance against these goals to ensure that an adequate, functioning credentialing system is in place or that progress is being made in this regard.

The Medical Staff Credentialing Audit

Unlike a financial audit, a medical staff credentialing audit or review is not something that must be performed on a yearly basis, although occasional reaudits can help to test and revalidate the system used by a hospital. The first credentialing audit, however, does far more. It establishes important benchmarks and guidance for all players in the hospital's credentialing system and provides the board with the objective, hard data and guidance it needs to play its proper role. Still, hospital directors may not be familiar with medical staff credentialing audits, and a bit more detail on what they are, how they work, and what they provide may be in order.

What Is a Medical Staff Credentialing Audit?

A medical staff credentialing audit is an independent review of a hospital's credentialing rules, forms, processes, documentation, and reports covering the four most critical credentialing areas: appointment, reappointment, corrective action, and internal decision reviews. The end product of an audit is a detailed management report stating the findings of the audit and listing specific recommendations for use by the medical staff, administration, and governing board for ensuring the effectiveness of the hospital's credentialing system. The audit thus meets one of the tree-clearing goals suggested in lesson four and suggests additional goals for future attainment.

Why Undertake a Medical Staff Credentialing Audit?

Breakdowns and flaws in the credentialing system are a major source of hospital and medical staff liability:

- Malpractice suits based on the hospital's negligence in appointing, reappointing, or failing to deal with inexpert physicians and other practitioners
- Federal antitrust suits based on the denial or termination of staff membership or clinical privileges
- State court suits by practitioners alleging injury in the credentialing process
- Failure of credentialing rules and processes to meet regulatory and other requirements

Equally as harmful, in many cases, are other difficulties caused by problem physicians who make it through the credentialing process:

- Financial loss caused by inappropriate utilization
- Serious and uncorrected problems relating to the quality of medical care

- Internal strife caused by disruptive practitioners
- Other peer review organization and accreditation problems

Effective credentialing systems keep inexpert and disruptive doctors from obtaining privileges, deal with problem practitioners with a minimum risk of liability, and serve to monitor ongoing performance to identify practitioners who need corrective assistance. The medical staff credentialing audit is designed to assist all players in the hospital credentialing process — medical staff, administration, and governance — in understanding the strengths and weaknesses of the hospital's credentialing system and to undertake an action plan to ensure the system's effectiveness. It can help take the mystery out of the credentialing system.

How Does a Medical Staff Credentialing Audit Work?

When a hospital undertakes a medical staff credentialing audit, an independent reviewer examines the rules, forms, processes, documentation, and reports used by the hospital in the credentialing of practitioners permitted to use the hospital's facilities. This examination covers appointment, reappointment, corrective action, and internal decision reviews.

A first step in the audit process is the identification and collection of documents, including application and reappointment forms, verification and reference forms and letters; checklists, minutes, and other reporting documents; bylaws; and representative files. Much of this material is reviewed prior to, and in preparation for, fieldwork at the hospital site.

During the site visit, further document review occurs. In addition, interviews take place with selected physicians, administrators and staff, and trustees involved in the hospital's credentialing system. At the end of the site visit, there is an exit interview with the administrator and key medical staff and board members.

The reviewer then prepares a written management report based on the examination. This confidential report contains detailed findings, observations, and recommendations — an action plan for use by the institution in updating the effectiveness of its credentialing system. The audit process ends with a presentation on-site to review the findings and recommendations of the report.

Good Performance for Liability Prevention

Early in this book, we noted that the law does not expect hospital directors to perform the job of management. However, it does expect directors to act in a reasonably prudent manner to ensure that things are done right. Directors are not expected to shadow professional managers and others to whom the board delegates functions, but they are expected to be reasonably well versed on matters of importance to the corporation and to have in place reasonably effective systems and safeguards that can be monitored to ensure performance.

The more important the operational area is to the success and well-being of a corporation, the more important this requirement is for the board. Hospital boards typically meet this requirement in finance, but fall short in medical staff credentialing. Hospitals and boards seldom face suits as a result of poor financial performance, but suits against hospitals and their directors do arise as a result of the failures of medical staff credentialing systems.

Boards looking for ways to improve their performance and prevent hospital and director liability in medical staff credentialing can and should look to success areas such as finance for lessons and guidance. They will find that success is a factor of time, knowledge, basic management processes, goals, and resource deployment and that employing these means will close the door on one important source of hospital director risk.

Chapter 6 looks at another area that can cause big trouble for hospital directors—corporate asset transactions such as those that take place in corporate restructuring, sales and mergers, diversification, and physician recruitment.

Chapter 6

Corporate Asset Transactions: Mergers, Sales, and Asset Transfers

When Good Buddy Hospital sold some of its valuable assets back in chapter 2, its directors got in trouble. Good Buddy is an entirely mythical hospital and the story is fabricated, but the outcome is very close to real. Transactions involving corporate assets probably form the one area of board involvement that generates the most damaging director liability in America today.

Most of the action occurs in business corporation settings and is readily understandable. When shareholders feel that their corporate directors have failed to obtain the maximum possible value in connection with the sale or merger of the corporation or the transfer of its assets, they get angry and they sue. After the Delaware Supreme Court decided the *Van Gorkom* case and the directors of Trans Union were found liable to the corporation for millions of dollars in damages, such suits increased in frequency. Even though many states have now adopted laws limiting director liability for breaches of the duty of care, suits alleging director malfeasance for failing to maximize stock value continue to be filed.

Things are a little different at the not-for-profit and public corporation end of the playing field. There are no angry shareholders here, and the action is less intense. But the rules can be complex and confusing, and when boards make mistakes, personal liability can be visited on the trustees who are at fault. Thus, when transactions involving corporate assets are brought to any board, it is time for the directors to sit up and take serious notice of what is going on.

Some Legal Principles

The authority of corporations to transfer or merge their assets and the procedures that must be followed are controlled by the state statutes under which the corporations are organized. In any sort of transaction, and particularly when a legal merger or major asset transfer is involved, boards should be aware of the statutory requirements and involve the hospital's attorney.

Public corporations, which hold their assets almost in a trust capacity for the public benefit, typically are under especially tight reign. Certain types of asset transfers may be prohibited, and others must meet strict valuation or competitive bidding rules. Federal rules concerning tax-exempt organizations may also apply, but these are seldom more stringent than the rules set by state law.

The rules governing not-for-profit corporations can vary significantly from state to state. These rules are found not only in the not-for-profit corporation statutes, but also in the state appellate court opinions that have been developed over the years. Although some of these are dated and arcane, they still apply to not-for-profit corporate activities.

The modern tendency of these state statutes and court opinions is to treat not-for-profit corporations very much as though they were business corporations and to allow them broad latitude. But some states cling to a notion rooted in the past—that not-for-profits bear a similarity to trusts and that certain fairly strict trust principles apply to their activities. Because most not-for-profit hospitals are tax-exempt under the Internal Revenue Code, federal tax rules may also apply to corporate asset transactions. Universally, not-for-profit corporation and federal tax-exemption laws prohibit the use of corporate assets for private use or gain.

The point of this recitation is that sales, mergers, and other asset transactions make up an amusement park for lawyers, with hoops to jump through and bells to ring. Fail to follow the rules and you pay a price. But enough legal mumbo jumbo! Let's see whether we can find some useful generalizations that can be applied here.

Asset Sales and Transfers to Private Parties

When not-for-profit hospitals sell, lease, loan, pledge, guarantee, invest in, or otherwise transfer any part of their assets to private parties, they must do so for fair value. The term *private party* in this case means any person or entity other than another not-for-profit or public corporation. There is a similarity between this requirement for not-for-profit corporations and the need to obtain maximum value in the for-profit setting: Failure can result in harm to the corporation and liability for the directors who approve the transaction.

What happens when this principle is violated? Clearly, the assets of the corporation are diminished. Furthermore, the state not-for-profit status of the corporation and its federal tax-exempt status are placed in jeopardy, and the loss of either status can be devastating. Directors who approve of the transaction or who, through inaction, allow it to take place are vulnerable in a number of ways.

As in the case of Good Buddy Hospital, the corporation can seek to recover from the directors the difference between the value of the transferred asset and the value received by the corporation. If the corporation loses its not-for-profit or tax-exempt status, the directors could be held personally liable for the damages suffered by the corporation. This is serious business, and there is no certainty that state director immunity laws will shield the directors from this risk.

Transfers to Other Not-for-Profit Entities

Not-for-profit corporations generally have greater freedom and latitude in sales and transfers (including legal mergers) involving other bona fide not-for-profit, tax-exempt organizations. This is because most states and federal tax rules are permissive when it comes to gifts and grants from one tax-exempt charitable corporation to another. In this setting, consideration in the form of fair value need not be exchanged in mergers or other activities in which assets are transferred. This permissiveness recognizes that no harm will result from the passage of an asset from the custody of one tax-exempt charity to another—that no private gain or benefit will occur.

But this permissiveness should not be overstated. Depending on the state law that applies to the transaction, there may be important conditions that must be met. It may be necessary that the not-for-profit corporations involved in the transaction be organized for similar purposes, that the giver and the taker, for example, both be hospitals or organizations engaged in the delivery and support of medical care. And it may be necessary that both corporations be organized under the laws of, and located in, the same state.

These requirements in some states flow from a view that not-for-profit (charitable) organizations are in the nature of trusts created under the laws of the state and recognized by the state for specific charitable purposes benefiting the people of the state. Gifts and grants to organizations that have different purposes or are located outside the state would violate the spirit of that trust and would therefore be *ultra vires*—beyond the authority granted to the corporation by the state. Directors who authorize or allow *ultra vires* conduct can be held liable for its consequences.

These considerations are of more than just passing interest in the current health care delivery environment. Hospital organizations consolidate across state lines and their managers routinely transfer funds and other assets from one corporation to another. Multiunit health care organizations form their various corporations for diverse purposes and move their assets around. In these settings boards must take care that routine transfers are not treated lightly and that legal attention is given to the requirements of applicable state laws.

Applying the Legal Principles

The reader may be wondering just how often hospital boards run up against situations involving asset transfers. Despite a relative frenzy of hospital merger activity in the for-profit and not-for-profit sectors, most hospital boards deal with mergers only once, if ever. And major asset sales or transfers are hardly a monthly event in most hospital organizations. Yet these and similar major events do occur, and countless smaller transactions also take place, as the following hypothetical examples illustrate.

Lease of Facilities

Three Counties District Hospital (TCDH) is a public hospital corporation organized under a special state statute authorizing the creation of public hospital districts. The boundaries of the district encompass three rural counties, and the board of commissioners for each county appoints four trustees to TCDH's board of directors. The hospital's administrator and the medical staff's president and president-elect serve ex officio.

The Public Hospital District Act under which TCDH is organized was adopted during the height of the Hill–Burton era, which was a long time ago, and has never been updated. Consequently, the act is terribly dated and restrictive. Although the hospital's service area is much broader than its boundaries, it is prevented by statute from operating satellite facilities outside the district. Severe restrictions also apply to its ability to recruit physicians, affiliate with other organizations, and do many other things thought necessary to improve its operations. County board interference in the operation of the hospital is also thought to be a problem and keeps the hospital from undertaking much-needed personnel reductions.

One day, the TCDH board had a great idea! It would create an all-new, not-for-profit hospital corporation, Three Counties Medical Center, Inc., and lease all of TCDH's grounds, facilities, and equipment to this new organization for 50 years at $1 a year. The new corporation would operate the facility as a private, not-for-profit hospital, free of the constraints of the Public Hospital District Act, and would be able to perform like a modern American hospital. It would even provide the same level of charity care as TCDH did in the past, so that everybody would be happy.

The idea seemed so perfect that it was undertaken immediately, with only a handful of the commissioner-appointed trustees dissenting. The new corporation was created, and its board was made up of the nondissenting trustees. Wearing their TCDH hats, the trustees directed TCDH's attorney, a state's attorney from one of the three counties, to draw up the lease to the new organization. The state's attorney refused, stating that district hospitals are prohibited from entering such leases under the state's Public Hospital District Act. The commissioners of all three counties also protested these activities.

Undaunted, the trustees put on their new medical center hats and hired their own attorney to draft a lease for approval by both organizations. When this was done, the new organization launched into business. The trustees formed a new medical staff, but refused membership to three doctors who had been on the staff of TCDH. They also hired as many of TCDH's employees as they felt were necessary to staff the hospital. The rest were left without jobs.

Here's what happened next. The three county boards filed suit, naming TCDH, the new medical center, and all of TCDH's assenting trustees and seeking to invalidate the lease to the new medical center as *ultra vires*. The suit also demanded restitution from the trustees for the damage caused to TCDH. Diverse suits were also filed by the doctors and employees who were not included on the new staff of the medical center. In various combinations, some of these suits named the trustees, some named the medical center, and some named TCDH. Things became so confused that all the suits were eventually consolidated into one legal action.

At trial the judge quickly concluded that the lease upon which all else hinged was, indeed, illegal. It didn't matter that the motives of the trustees were pure, that their actions would have led to improvements in health care delivery, or that other states had amended their public hospital laws to permit similar transactions.

The state statute that formed the basis for all corporate actions by Three Counties District Hospital stated in black and white that leases of hospital district assets "other than in the ordinary course of business" were prohibited. The judge found that the lease was not in the ordinary course of business. Thus, the lease was voided, and the grounds, equipment, and facilities were returned to TCDH to resume hospital operations. And the responsible trustees were removed from the TCDH board.

What about the remaining debris? All of the aggrieved doctors and employees were returned to their former status. The damages they suffered and the damages suffered by TCDH were calculated and assessed against the former trustees whose *ultra vires* acts were the root cause. Because they were aware that they were acting in violation of the law and yet did so intentionally, they were not protected by state director immunity laws.

Moral of the story: In transfer of asset transactions, know what the law requires and don't take it lightly.

Physician Recruitment

In chapter 3, we spent some time asking questions about possible board criminal liability in connection with illegal physician "incentive" programs at Stichem Community Hospital. We did this, in part, because violation of Medicare fraud and abuse rules is a major issue in physician recruitment and incentive programs. The other big issue in this arena is violation of federal tax and state corporation rules regarding private benefit and private inurement in tax-exempt, not-for-profit hospitals. If a not-for-profit hospital pays doctors money to admit patients, it's guilty of Medicare fraud. If it pays doctors money for no reason at all, it breaks corporation law and tax rules and can lose its tax-exempt and not-for-profit status. Both types of payment are asset transactions that can cause personal liability problems for hospital directors.

Now here are some other things that happened at Stichem. In order to attract more new doctors to the hospital, Stichem's administrator devised a multifaceted program and presented it to the board for review and approval. Everyone knows that doctors need offices and that if those offices are close by, the hospital will get a good share of the doctors' patient admissions. Part one of the administrator's plan was to build a lavish medical arts building equipped with a sports fitness center.

Offices in the center would be rented to doctors at ridiculously low rents that bore no relationship to market rates or the cost of building and maintaining the facility. With an indoor lap pool, jogging track, two tennis courts, and other court facilities, the sports center would be open only to doctors on the hospital's medical staff, hospital trustees, and top administrative personnel. There would be no cost for this privilege.

Part two of the plan would provide loans to any new, non-hospital-based doctor who joined Stichem's medical staff. It would work like this: Each doctor would receive one check for $50,000 upon being accepted to the medical staff and another check for $50,000 on the anniversary date of his or her appointment. There would be no note or security for the loan. It would be given with the understanding that it would be paid back when it was convenient for the doctor.

The administrator had recently learned that any attempt to tie the elements of this plan to hospital admissions would be a felony under the Medicare fraud and abuse statutes, and so no admitting requirement was incorporated into the plan. Stichem's trustees would normally have thought that the administrator had gone berserk with this giveaway plan, but past performance with other goofy schemes had been excellent, and the trustees were intrigued by the concept of the sports center. Thus, they approved and authorized funding for the plan out of cash reserves earned in better times and an old designated fund account. The designated fund account resulted from a substantial grant made many years earlier for the care of the blind and elderly, "like the people who would be served by the new physicians" (the administrator said).

Whether this scheme worked to build hospital admissions doesn't really matter here. What does matter is that a few years later two things happened. First, auditors from the Internal Revenue Service stopped by to conduct a routine audit of this tax-exempt organization. Second, the grandchildren of Pa Stichem, the person who had made the grant of funds for the care of the blind and elderly, learned that their lost inheritance had been used in part to build a private health spa. Boy, were they mad.

The tax auditors were not pleased by what they found either, but they were motivated. They concluded that hospital funds had been used—and used in abundance—for the private benefit and enjoyment of doctors, trustees, and administrators of the hospital and that the hospital had sought and received nothing of comparable value in return. They recommended that the tax-exempt status of the hospital be withdrawn retroactive to the start of the giveaway program.

This was done, and back taxes and penalties were levied on the hospital corporation. Information was also turned over to the U.S. Department of Justice for possible criminal investigation of the hospital, and tax audits of the doctors, trustees, and administrators who had received so much benefit from the hospital were undertaken to see whether they had underreported their incomes.

The Stichem kin tried to sue the hospital and the board for the inappropriate use of funds that had been granted to the hospital by their grandfather, and after having their suit dismissed for lack of standing, they enlisted the support of the state's attorney general. A new suit was brought by the attorney general seeking restitution from the trustees to the hospital of all of the moneys given away or inappropriately spent. This suit was successful and also resulted in court-ordered replacement of the board. The new board then sued the old board to seek payment of damages suffered by the corporation due to its loss of tax-exempt status. This suit was also successful.

In all of these suits the old trustees tried to invoke the immunity protections granted by the state's corporation statute. But in all cases the judges found that the trustees had acted with reckless indifference to their duty of care and that by benefiting personally from the use of the health spa they had violated their duty of loyalty as well. What an ugly story, but, oh, the truth it holds!

Sale or Merger of the Hospital Corporation

These are only stories, however, and the outcome doesn't have to be so bleak. The trustees of Tiny General Hospital, for example, pretty well agreed that the future viability of the place required some sort of alliance with a larger, more resilient organization. Tiny General's corporation was not-for-profit and tax-exempt, organized with the corporate purpose of providing hospital and related health care services to the residents of Tinytown and the surrounding area.

In a neighboring state was HealthMega, a not-for-profit, tax-exempt hospital holding company that was strong, dynamic, and growing. HealthMega owned or controlled five hospitals, outpatient centers, nursing homes, and retirement centers providing a continuum of care, and it was looking for acquisition candidates.

The trustees of Tiny were drawn to HealthMega, and vice versa. They thought HealthMega's mission, represented by its slogan, "Where compassion makes our day!" corresponded to its own, "They call us Tiny, but we're big at heart!" And they thought that HealthMega would do a good job as custodian of Tiny's resources. So discussions began in earnest concerning some sort of coming together.

The trustees of Tiny realized that this coming together would result in giving up significant control — maybe total control — of the hospital, but they didn't mind. They just wanted to ensure some immediate benefit for their hospital. They wanted HealthMega to undertake some needed capital improvements to the hospital, which Tiny lacked the vigor to accomplish on its own, and they wanted to fund and continue to control the Tiny Hospital Foundation so that they could support certain hospital programs and maintain some involvement in hospital affairs.

HealthMega had the megabucks to undertake the improvements and was not averse to transferring some amount, to be negotiated, to the foundation. In essence, the two parties had the makings of a deal. What they needed was a form to accomplish the deal, and they found it in what they characterized as a "sale" of Tiny General Hospital, Inc., to HealthMega. The consequence of using this form was that Tiny, Inc., would continue as an identifiable corporate entity rather than being merged into HealthMega and disappearing. The reason for the use of this form is not important here.

This transaction is referred to as a "sale" in quotation marks, because, in reality, not-for-profit corporations can't be sold. There are no shareholders. Nobody owns them, and one cannot sell what one does not own. Still, the transaction looked like a sale, because in return for gaining control over Tiny, HealthMega would be making commitments and paying other consideration. In any event, the trustees of Tiny came to think of and treat the transaction as a sale in form if not in fact.

One of Tiny's trustees was very concerned about director liability issues and had followed the plights of boards as reported in a weekly business magazine for several years. One thing had become ingrained in this trustee's head, and that is that someone would sue the breeches off corporate trustees if they failed to get maximum value in the sale of the corporation or business for which they were responsible. The trustee was frustrated and angry that Tiny's board had not commissioned an expensive valuation study and that the board seemed willing to "give away the corporation," in the trustee's words, for mere promises and a contribution to the foundation. "The amounts involved here don't come anywhere near approximating the value of our corporation," said the trustee, "and we all stand liable if we let this deal go down like this."

These were scary words. However, the remainder of the board wasn't sure whether the trustee was on target, and so it asked Tiny General's attorney for an opinion. The attorney was pretty sure about the answer, but undertook appropriately extensive research to be on the safe side. Here's what the research showed.

Under the laws of the state in which Tiny was incorporated, not-for-profit organizations such as Tiny were authorized to make gifts and grants to other not-for-profit corporations that were organized for similar purposes. The law and state appellate cases were silent as to whether such transfers of assets could be made to organizations, such as HealthMega, incorporated in other states, but two things seemed to favor a positive view. One was that many such transfers had been made openly by not-for-profit corporations in the state and had never been challenged. To the extent that practice makes the law (where the law is otherwise silent), practice in this case would seem to condone interstate transfers between not-for-profit corporations with similar purposes.

The second was that the transaction between Tiny and HealthMega wouldn't really result in a transfer of assets by Tiny. As we said earlier, although it might look like a sale, it wasn't one. There would be a change in the control or stewardship of the corporation, but the corporation would continue to own the assets. The only transfer of assets that would take place was the one involving HealthMega's donation of funds to Tiny Hospital Foundation, and that, in the main, was HealthMega's problem if it was a problem at all.

This well-researched and reasoned opinion failed, however, to please Tiny's doubting trustee, who remained convinced that the transaction had the potential of becoming another *Smith v. Van Gorkom*,[1] but that just goes to show that reasonable people with the same facts are capable of coming to different conclusions. The transaction was consummated with one opposing vote, and the parties lived happily ever after.

Indeed, the cast in this story did almost everything it should have done. The doubting trustee raised the doubt rather than sitting on it. The board instructed counsel for the hospital to provide a considered opinion rather than stonewalling the one trustee who was out of synch. And the doubting trustee, still unpersuaded, cast a vote of conscience rather than going along with the gang. One thing is sure, if the doubting trustee was right, that dissenting vote, duly recorded in the corporate minutes, was the surest possible ticket to freedom from liability.

If Tiny's board had one failing, it was one that you didn't read about above. The board took the strength and capabilities of HealthMega on faith rather than undertaking a diligent review. We'll assume that HealthMega, in fact, had no major weaknesses, that it was able to meet its commitments, and that it maintained Tiny General as a viable community hospital. But what if this hadn't been the case? This is a question that shouldn't have to be asked. Reasonably prudent directors would make sure of the answer before entering into the transaction.

Funding For-Profit Affiliates

Straight Arrow Hospital always tried to do the right thing, and so when it set up a special program for physician recruitment and decided to buy a pizza franchise, it established two separate new business corporations. The reasons for following this approach were made clear by Straight Arrow's lawyer: By operating physician recruitment through a for-profit affiliate, the private benefit and private inurement problems present in the not-for-profit, tax-exempt corporation setting could be avoided. By operating the new Pizza Power! franchise through a for-profit affiliate, problems involving tax-exempt organization limitations on unrelated business income would also be eliminated. These sounded like good reasons to Straight Arrow's board, and so it approved these actions and authorized initial funding for the new corporations.

In the case of the physician recruitment corporation, named SAH, Inc., Straight Arrow purchased all capital shares for $100,000 and made a loan of $250,000 secured by an open-ended note. Straight Arrow's board also named three of its members to serve as the directors of SAH, Inc. In the case of Pizza Power! the plan was a little different. Because the pizza idea was brought to Straight Arrow by one of its most loyal internists, Straight Arrow agreed that it would participate as a preferred stock shareholder, with an option to convert its preferred shares into 51 percent ownership of the voting common stock.

Straight Arrow bought its preferred shares for $750,000. The internist and a few other physician investors bought the original issue of common stock for $20,000 and elected themselves directors of Pizza Power!(SA), Inc. Straight Arrow's board was told that this arrangement would result in preferential payment of dividends to the hospital corporation and, if necessary, could be converted into a controlling interest in Pizza Power!

SAH, Inc., hired a small staff and embarked on an aggressive program of physician recruitment and medical practice acquisition. After five months it requested another loan of $250,000 from Straight Arrow, which was authorized by Straight Arrow's board on the same terms as before. Over the next two years another $1.5 million was loaned to SAH, Inc., by Straight Arrow's administrator without specific board authorization. The amounts transferred were duly recorded in Straight Arrow's financial records, however, and showed as an asset on its financial statement.

The directors of SAH, Inc., knew about the additional transfers, and because they sat as directors of Straight Arrow Hospital, they also knew that there had been no Straight Arrow board action to authorize the loans. None of Straight Arrow's trustees was too concerned about this situation, however. After all, SAH, Inc., had been set up only to meet legal form requirements so that physician recruiting could take place. So they let the matter slide and never sought an accounting of how the funds had been used or when the loans would be paid back.

If they had, they would have found that all of the money invested in and loaned to SAH, Inc., had been paid out to cover operating expenses, purchase medical practices, and make loans to doctors for diverse reasons. Whether funds loaned to the for-profit SAH, Inc., by not-for-profit Straight Arrow would ever be paid back would have been found to be questionable, and there was absolutely no chance that Straight Arrow would ever be paid dividends on its equity investment. SAH, Inc., simply was not set up or organized to make money. It was a front.

Pizza Power! built its pizza palace in the parking lot of a shopping center with only small cost overruns and opened for business. To everyone's surprise, the business far exceeded expectations in its first 18 months of operation and paid Straight Arrow its full 10 percent dividend. Remaining post-tax profits were paid as dividends to the doctors holding the common stock. They got $100,000 on their $20,000 investment.

But, alas, business then dried up. First, there was a series of salmonella attacks that twice shut the pizza palace down and caused pizza lovers to look elsewhere for their pepperoni and cheese. Then, formidable new competition sprang up in a new shopping center a quarter of a mile away. After six months of losses, Straight Arrow Hospital converted its preferred shares to common stock and took over control of Pizza Power!(SA), Inc.

After six more months of losses, the restaurant was closed, and the facility was sold for $150,000 to a group of doctors planning to open a hot dog franchise. After Pizza Power!'s debts were paid, the corporation was liquidated, and the remaining $40,800 dollars was divided among the holders of common stock, which came to $20,800 for Straight Arrow Hospital (on its original investment of $750,000) and $20,000 for the internist and his friends. Straight Arrow's board vowed never again to get the hospital involved in such a fiasco.

What happened next? Nothing, really. Well, almost nothing. The Internal Revenue Service did conduct a routine and somewhat careless audit of Straight Arrow Hospital, Inc., but failed to delve into the asset transactions just discussed. A concurrent audit at neighboring Stichem Community Hospital had diverted the Internal Revenue Service's resources.

However, unbelievably expensive tax counsel retained by Straight Arrow's board at the time of the audit gave the directors a good scare by telling them that the investment actions they had taken could have resulted in the loss of the organization's tax-exempt status. SAH, Inc., was just a front for indirectly making fund transfers that Straight Arrow was prohibited by law from making directly. And the structure of the Pizza Power! investment, an asset transaction intended to produce income for the hospital, inadvertently used tax-exempt funds to provide undeserved enrichment to private individuals who had taken on only minimal risk. In sum, Straight Arrow's board permitted the kind of activity that could have gotten the directors in deep trouble. But they were lucky.

Asset Transfers to Affiliated Corporations

Finally, we turn to asset transfers made by tax-exempt, not-for-profit hospital corporations to their parent and other affiliated tax-exempt, not-for-profit corporations—routine practice in today's corporately restructured hospital world. Under federal tax and state not-for-profit corporation law, these transfers—really gifts and grants—generally are permitted. Their occurrence is so commonplace that even the issues raised earlier in this chapter—those dealing with transfers across state lines and to corporations lacking similar purposes—typically are overlooked. Indeed, many legal experts would question, verbally at least, whether these issues merit any attention today.

One aspect of these intercorporate transfers that unquestionably deserves the attention of hospital directors, however, is their effect on the granting or donor corporation and the responsibility of corporate directors to act independently in the best interests of the corporation. For the fact is that these intercorporate asset transfers often are not freely donated by the trustees of the donor corporations; they are directed from above by the parent corporation.

You may recall that in chapter 3 Good Buddy Hospital was taken over by a Catholic religious order. We'll call the order the Sisters of Mt. O . . . and its hospital holding company Mt. O . . . Nationwide Services, Inc. (MONSI). MONSI appointed the trustees to the board of Good Buddy and could also remove the trustees at its discretion. It also retained power over Good Buddy's budget, assets, bylaws, planning, and the like.

In short, though the Good Buddy board could *take* independent action, it couldn't necessarily *effect* independent action. If the trustees attempted independent action that displeased MONSI, they would be, in a word, "gone." That's why it was said in chapter 3 that "when corporate [MONSI] speaks, the sponsored institutions [that is, Good Buddy] are expected to jump." This was the rule of the game, and the trustees of Good Buddy Hospital understood and accepted it. They did their best to operate within this limited scope of authority.

MONSI operated hospitals all over the United States. Financially, some of them did very poorly, some of them (like Good Buddy) did all right, and some of them did very well. Some of the hospitals, especially the poor performers, were badly in need of capital improvements, and MONSI orchestrated a massive tax-exempt bond sale to provide funds.

Of course, the poor performers could never have qualified for credit, and so in order to provide collateral and security for the bond issue MONSI enlisted the participation of all the hospitals in its system. Each hospital corporation under the sisters' sponsorship and MONSI's control was instructed to approve and execute bond documents that guaranteed payment of the bonds and pledged the assets and revenues of the corporation as security in the case of a default.

Good Buddy Hospital was not slated to receive any of the proceeds of the bond issue, and some of its trustees had misgivings about placing the hospital corporation's assets on the line. In addition to putting the assets at risk, these trustees were concerned that by doing so Good Buddy would lose its own private access to debt capital should a need arise in the future. Nonetheless, Good Buddy's trustees performed the required acts as instructed. The corporation pledged its assets and agreed to guarantee payment of the bonds, both classic forms of asset transactions.

At about the same time, one of MONSI's inner-city hospitals, located not very distant from Good Buddy, experienced severe shortages of operating capital. Part of the sisters' mission was to serve and minister to the poor, and MONSI was not about to let this hospital go down the tube. Because Good Buddy "shared a kindred spirit and sphere of interest" with the destitute hospital and had $2 million of hard-earned cash in the bank, MONSI suggested that the Good Buddy board donate $1.5 million to ease the crunch. Again, the trustees of Good Buddy were not crazy about making this intercorporate transfer, but what choice did they have? They authorized it and received a pat on the back for doing a good thing.

The reader can see, perhaps, where this story is headed. The pressures of decreased hospital utilization and decreased reimbursement put a terrible squeeze on the systemwide revenues of the MONSI hospitals. To meet debt service, Good Buddy Hospital and the other obligated hospitals in the system were required to pay ever-increasing amounts of their operating income. Systemwide operations faltered. Eventually, there was a default on the bonds, and the assets pledged by Good Buddy fell to the creditors. Good Buddy went into receivership and eventually closed.

Doctors on Good Buddy's medical staff and the folks in Good Buddy's hometown were outraged by the loss of their only hospital facility. The local paper published an investigative report on the episode and in an accompanying editorial made the following comments:

PROSECUTE GOOD BUDDY CULPRITS

It is difficult to conceive of how the trustees of Good Buddy Hospital, local citizens who were entrusted with the custody of and expected to safeguard one of our most important community resources, could have acted in such an irresponsible and foolish manner.

They literally gave away, with no strings attached and with no return of benefit, more than a million dollars — money taken from our citizenry! — to an urban hospital with no connection to our community. Worse, they pledged the assets and revenues of our hospital in a risky capital venture that never produced a single benefit for the hospital or our town.

Good Buddy, indeed! These trustees have done the greatest disservice imaginable, and the attorney general of this state, who is empowered to police such irresponsible conduct, should use the facts uncovered in our investigation to prosecute these individuals to the fullest extent of the law.

The attorney general did prosecute the trustees, and a jury found them culpable of breaching their duty of care to the corporation. They were ordered to pay the defunct corporation millions of dollars, moneys needed to pay the corporation's debts and reopen the hospital. The defenses used by the trustees—that they were protected by the state's statute granting certain immunity from liability and that their actions were excusable because they lacked the authority to act independently in the best interests of the corporation—were found to be invalid.

The verdict was appealed all the way to the state's supreme court, where it was upheld. Concerning the defense that the trustees lacked authority to act independently, the supreme court opinion read something like this:

> We find this contention that the trustees lacked authority to act independently to be wholly lacking in merit, for it demonstrates a fundamental misunderstanding of the role and duty of corporate directors under the laws of our state. Our statute holds the corporate directors *solely* responsible for managing the affairs of the corporation, and our common law holds that these directors have a fiduciary duty to carry out this responsibility in the best interests of the corporation, and the corporation alone.
>
> The defendants here would have us believe that they could meet neither this statutory responsibility nor this fiduciary duty because of the "control structure" put in place by Mt. O . . . Nationwide Services, Inc. It is true that the directors could be removed if their decisions did not please their master, and it is also true that the master retained powers to such a degree that it could veto any action of Good Buddy Hospital, Inc. But these circumstances do not relieve the directors of their burden to abide by the legal requirements of this state.
>
> The directors here had no impediment to independent action. There was no "gun to their heads." They did not have to do what the master ordered if they believed that the ordered action was contrary to the best interests of the corporation. Each director was free to resign from the board if the ordered action violated his or her judgment of what was best. Each director was free to vote his or her mind, with the only consequence being dismissal from the board if the master was angered.
>
> Had the directors here exercised independent judgment by casting and recording votes against the action ordered by the master, the reasons for this suit against them might never have arisen. Had the directors withdrawn from or caused their own dismissal from the board rather than serve as mere proxy bearers, it is the master, rather than the defendants here, who would have been held accountable for the ills suffered by the corporation.

Moral of the story: Directors must exercise independent judgment, and this responsibility cannot be abdicated. Just as it was in childhood, if something bad happens because of what you did, you can't get away with it because someone bigger told you to do it. In the modern hospital setting there may be many instances in which a corporate parent directs action by a subsidiary board. When these directives relate to asset transactions (or other major corporate actions), great caution and independent judgment should be exercised.

Exercising Proper Stewardship

Indeed, safeguarding the assets of the corporation and using them in the best interests of the corporation is what the corporate director's job is all about. In the nonprofit hospital sector, where the corporation functions as a charity, this is especially important. Although it is stylish for nonprofit hospital organizations to organize themselves and act like their for-profit counterparts, the public, its elected officials, and the courts may be less inclined to go along.

It is a good bet that the future will see increasing instances in which hospital corporation asset transactions, like the ones described in this chapter, are called into question, and the directors who approved them will feel the heat of the spotlight. In this setting prudent directors will be best served by remembering and exercising their stewardship role as caretakers and custodians of the corporation's assets. By doing so, they will have gone a long way toward preventing their own personal liability.

In the next chapter we look at two additional areas of director risk and summarize risk prevention actions that hospital boards can take.

☐ *Reference*

1. Smith v. Van Gorkom, 488 A.2d 858.

Chapter 7

Conflicts, Compliance, and Board Risk Management

Conflicts of interest and the failure of boards or groups of directors to abide by rules of the organization or the state of incorporation constitute another important area of director risk. This chapter deals with these two subjects in greater detail and provides some pointers that boards may find useful when they look for ways to manage the risk of director liability.

Director Conflicts of Interest

In chapter 3, we discussed the legal fiduciary duty of loyalty, one of the three legal duties that apply to directors of all corporations. The duty of loyalty requires that directors avoid competing with the corporation, usurping its business opportunities, profiteering from insider information, or otherwise acting in conflict with the best interests of the corporation. Hospital boards were urged to devise and draft conflict-of-interest policies and procedures to help hospital directors and boards understand the requirement and avoid inadvertent conflicts that could get directors in deep trouble.

People who serve on hospital boards—community members, businesspeople, doctors, other professionals, bankers, corporate managers, religious, just about anybody—will frequently find themselves facing some kind of *duality of interest* with the hospital corporation. Some aspect of the hospital's activities will intersect with some aspect of their personal activities in a way that makes it possible for conflicts between personal and corporate interests to arise. Duality of interests is a fact of life in all corporate settings that, in most cases, is recognized and tolerated by the law.

Still, in some public corporation settings, certain dualities of interest are thought to create such a strong potential for disloyal conduct that persons who suffer the duality are prohibited by state statute from serving on public hospital boards. And beyond these specific cases, directors are often unclear concerning their proper conduct when dualities and conflicts with corporate interests arise. Hospital board conflict-of-interest policies provide an opportunity to describe the hard-and-fast legal rules found in the statutes of the state in which the hospital corporation is organized and to provide helpful general guidance for directors as they try to sort out their personal conduct on the board.

Board Conflict-of-Interest Policies

Board conflict-of-interest policies state the philosophy of the corporation concerning conflicts, provide needed definitions, and describe the policy's scope of coverage, disclosure requirements, and prohibited activities. Although such policies can follow any number of formats, the following considerations all require attention.

Examining State Law on Conflict Policy

The starting point in devising any corporate board conflict policy is the statute under which the hospital corporation is organized. Frequently, these statutes state the jurisdiction's public policy concerning conflicts and list procedures that must be followed by individual directors and boards when a potential director conflict presents itself. When these statutory requirements are met, directors will be presumed by the law not to have engaged in a conflict that would violate the legal duty of loyalty.

Not all corporation law statutes embody provisions dealing with conflicts, however. In jurisdictions where this is the case, it is necessary to go to the state's common law and seek whatever guidance can be found in appellate court decisions. This may not be as difficult as it seems, because director conflicts historically have generated lots of litigation and the courts have had ample opportunity to set guidelines on what constitutes permissible or wrongful conduct.

Adopting a Written Conflict Policy

State rules, whether statutory or common-law, should form the core of any conflict policy adopted by a hospital board. Boards may, however, wish to adopt rules that are broader or more stringent than those found in state law. For example, state laws generally do not require that corporations adopt written policies regarding conflicts. As suggested here, however, this is something that boards should do.

Also, except in the public corporation setting, state laws generally do not bar individuals who do business with the corporation from serving on its board. Hospital directors may decide on their own, however, that the board is better and more safely served by excluding individuals who make some or all of their living through the sale of goods or services to the organization.

Including the Activities of Nondirectors in Policy

State law conflict requirements may not extend beyond corporation directors. Hospital boards may feel, however, that their conflict rules and procedures should apply beyond the directors and include the activities of spouses, children, and other members of directors' families. Boards may also decide to extend the corporation's conflict policy and procedures to key employees, medical staff officers, volunteers, and others whose personal conflicts could injure the corporation.

Broadening the Definition of Conflict

State conflict-of-interest statutes and case law attempt to define the kinds of conduct that constitute a conflict that violates the duty of loyalty to the corporation. In the business corporation setting the law traditionally has condoned a broad range of activities, and the trend of the law in the not-for-profit setting is to follow this lead. Hospital boards may wish to employ stricter standards in their own conflict policies than those embodied in state law.

Incorporating Policy into Corporate Bylaws

If state law does not require that corporate bylaws contain a conflict-of-interest provision, hospital boards may wish to use this approach on their own initiative. There are two points of view regarding this practice. On the one hand, placing the corporation's conflict policy in the bylaws may require cumbersome action and may make needed amendments difficult to effect. On the other hand, placement in the bylaws raises the policy's level of importance and force, and when placed in the bylaws, the policy can provide for removal of a director who intentionally violates its directives.

Procedures for Disclosing and Handling Conflicts of Interest

Again, state law is the starting point for determining what kind of procedures should be required of hospital boards and directors in disclosing and dealing with conflicts. With regard to disclosure, however, two approaches are open to corporations. The conflict policy of the board can rely on directors to come forward and make disclosures on their own when such disclosure is required or appropriate. Alternatively, the policy can require the use of a periodic disclosure questionnaire. An American Hospital Association publication cited later in this chapter contains a sample questionnaire that boards can use as a model for their own.

The voluntary approach is unquestionably less burdensome for directors and the corporation, but it is probably less effective than the periodic disclosure questionnaire approach. Use of the periodic and usually annual survey process serves to provide a regular reminder to directors and other covered persons regarding the contents and requirements of the corporation's policy. The approach also generates a greater level of introspection on the part of directors and others as they think about and prepare their answers. Finally, the approach provides for revelation of dualities of interest that could give rise to serious conflicts before such conflicts arise and helps everybody better steer their course.

Periodic disclosure questionnaires, however, never can be made sufficiently comprehensive to uncover every possible or meaningful duality of interest. For example, the trustee of a hospital that has always employed its own administrator may have a sibling, child, or spouse high in the control structure of a hospital management company that is not active in the area, and the director may not view this situation as creating any duality of interest. This seems fair enough. Then one day the hospital administrator retires, and the board decides to consider use of a management company rather than hire a new chief executive. Suddenly, there is a meaningful duality of interest that could interfere with the trustee's loyalty to the corporation.

In this sort of situation it is not enough for the trustee to rely on a periodic disclosure questionnaire to meet the duty to disclose. This trustee should come forward independently, let the other members of the board know about the duality of interest, and abide by the corporation's policy concerning a continued role in this specific board matter.

Further Guidance for Conflict-of-Interest Policies

In 1975, the American Hospital Association prepared and first published an excellent set of guidelines concerning conflicts of interest entitled *Resolution of Conflicts of Interest in Health Care Institutions.*[1] For over a decade, this publication has served as the basis for actions taken by many hospital boards in America. It is still available from the association.

Many state and regional hospital associations have also prepared materials dealing with the subject of conflicts, including policy and procedure statements, and they should be consulted by hospital boards wishing to adopt or update conflict policies and procedures for their corporations. But in all cases there must also be a careful review of current state conflict-of-interest law concerning corporate directors. This law changes from time to time, and boards should take care to ensure periodically that the practices employed by their hospital corporations are attuned to the current state legal standards.

A Final Caution on Conflicts

Board conflict policies and procedures are good tools, but they certainly aren't foolproof. Boards can adopt them, implement them, and monitor their results, but only individual directors through their personal conduct can ensure that wrongful and damaging conflicts never arise. In most private settings the law tolerates a wide degree of business dealings between directors and the corporation, but this is still an area in which directors may go astray.

The surest way for a hospital director to avoid exposure to a legal claim based on a conflict of interest — and the attention, expense, and embarrassment such claims invariably cause — is fairly simple and direct. Although state law may countenance the practice, don't buy things from or sell things to your corporation. If you must buy or sell, get off or stay off the board.

Compliance with Corporation Law and Corporate Rules

Hospital directors can be sued when they fail to abide by the prohibitions, methods, and procedures for doing things stated in corporate bylaws and articles of incorporation and in the law under which the corporation is organized. The need to comply with these rules was described in chapter 3 as part of the duty of obedience. One would think that directors would understand this need and that lawsuits in this area would be rare. Yet the opposite is true. Although damages in successful suits in this area are usually less severe than in suits involving corporate assets and conflicts of interest, this is still an area of proper concern.

In chapter 3, we also noted that much of the litigation involving violations of corporation law and corporate rules concerning methods and procedures are among the directors themselves and frequently involve control issues. Let's look at some of the specific rule areas to better understand what is involved here.

Amendments to Articles of Incorporation

An organization's articles of incorporation, or charter, is one of two legal documents that can state important rules governing the control of the corporation. The articles are especially important in business corporations, where they may state the rules concerning shareholder rights. Amendments to the charter can result in the gain or loss of control or important rights for shareholders, members of not-for-profit corporations, or board members.

The methods for amending the articles of incorporation are governed by state statutes, corporate bylaws, or the articles themselves. State statutes typically describe the process that must be used for amendment if the matter is not dealt with in the articles or bylaws, and they also set certain minimal requirements that must be met when amendment procedures are dealt with in these documents. The rules concerning amendments prescribed in the state statutes are supreme. Those contained in the articles are second in supremacy, and those of the bylaws are last.

Poorly drafted or outdated corporate documents can result in conflicts with statutory requirements or among themselves, and resulting disagreements about interpretation can lead to disputes among directors vying for control or seeking other advantageous changes. Sometimes director factions find it convenient simply to ignore the amendment rules in order to get amendments they want or ignore the rules through inadvertence, and these actions can also result in director litigation.

Other Rule Areas of Potential Risk

The foregoing narrative may provide the reader with more (or less) information than is desired, but it gives an idea of the motives or circumstances sometimes involved and of the legal complexity of the subject. From here on, however, we'll just list corporation law and corporate rule areas that can give rise to director lawsuits:

- Amendments to corporate bylaws, for much the same reason described in the preceding section
- Disputes concerning quorums for meetings
- Disputes involving the plurality needed or received for board action
- Election or removal of directors and officers
- Meeting notice requirements and disputes concerning the conduct of meetings or the right or failure to call meetings
- Approvals needed for mergers and consolidations, disposition of assets, and dissolution

In many "restructured" not-for-profit hospital corporations with a single, controlling corporate member, the articles of incorporation or, more frequently, the bylaws of the hospital corporation list a number of powers usually exercised by a corporate board that are retained by the member. These retained powers usually relate to organization, control, and financial issues and may cover planning and ethical issues as well. Hospital trustees who grow tired of the "corporate" yoke and attempt to infringe on these retained powers also set themselves up as prime targets for lawsuits undertaken by, or at the instigation of, the parent member.

Litigation Prevention

In most cases, directors of hospital corporations clearly have the means to avoid being drawn into litigation over the failure to follow the state corporation law and corporate rules listed here. The key is to be familiar with the rules and to obey them.

Ensuring Familiarity with Corporate Documents

Hospital directors should all have copies of the current articles of incorporation and bylaws of the corporation so that they can familiarize themselves with the contents. Although these corporate documents can seem tedious, directors should read them from time to time and have any questions about them answered to their satisfaction. To do less falls short of reasonably prudent conduct. Reasonable prudence also requires that the corporate rules should be available at all meetings and consulted when questions arise about their application.

Ensuring Conformity of Corporate Documents

Directors should also satisfy themselves from time to time that the rules contained in the corporation's charter and bylaws are not in conflict with themselves or the requirements found in the state corporation law controlling the corporation. This is lawyer's work, and the hospital attorney's review and opinion should be sought.

Handling Significant Corporate Undertakings

When significant and out-of-the-ordinary activities are undertaken by the corporation—such as a merger; a bond issue; the sale, lease, or granting of major corporate assets; the establishment of a new corporation; or the dissolution of a subsidiary corporation—directors should also enlist legal counsel to ensure that state statutory requirements, as well as those of the corporation's charter and bylaws, are being met.

Determining Other Statutory Rules Governing Directors

State corporation laws also prohibit and hold directors personally liable for certain actions. Some of these, such as the prohibition found in some states on the authorization of loans by not-for-profit corporations to directors and officers, are readily understandable. Other prohibitions, however, relate to more arcane subjects, such as authorizing the continuation of business in the corporate name after dissolution. The rules vary from state to state. They also vary among different kinds of corporations in any given state.

Hospital directors have two means of finding out about these prohibitions so that inadvertent violation does not occur. They can read the statute under which their corporation is organized, or they can instruct the administrator to obtain a written description of these laws for them. The latter approach seems more attractive.

Risk Management for Hospital Directors

Up to this point we've reviewed subject areas that tend to pose the greatest risk of personal liability for hospital directors. As we end this chapter, we shift the focus slightly to look at or summarize actions that individual directors and boards as a whole can take to limit their exposure to liability. These hospital board risk management strategies include the recording of votes in the corporate minutes and a small but important bill of rights for hospital directors.

The Need to Record Votes

Directors act through their votes, and their votes are what get them into trouble or keep trouble from the door. How those votes are recorded in the minutes of meetings can be just as important as the votes themselves.

This matter of votes and how they are recorded is dealt with by the corporation laws of most states. State laws, of course, vary, and hospital directors who fail to educate themselves about the law that applies to their votes make a big mistake. The Illinois rule for not-for-profit corporations is illustrative:

> A director of a corporation who is present at a meeting of its board of directors at which action on any corporate matter is taken is conclusively presumed to have assented to the action taken unless his or her dissent or abstention is entered in the minutes of the meeting or unless he or she files his or her written dissent or abstention to such action with the person acting as the secretary of the meeting before the adjournment thereof or forwards such dissent or abstention by registered or certified mail to the secretary of the corporation immediately after the adjournment of the meeting. Such right to dissent or abstain does not apply to a director who voted in favor of such action.[2]

Director beware! Unless you actually voice your nay or abstention, you will be counted among the directors who approved an action. If you were at the meeting but your no vote or abstention does not show in the minutes, you will be presumed to have voted in favor of the action. Those minutes are important. If you believe in your soul that an action considered by the board is wrong, you must express your belief by your vote, and you must ensure that the way you voted is properly reflected in the minutes of the meeting.

Other Risk Management Guidance

Chapter 8 of *Malpractice Prevention and Liability Control for Hospitals* by Orlikoff and Vanagunas describes a risk management program that boards might consider as a means of reducing director liability. This program is composed of three steps:

1. Determining potential liability exposure
2. Assessing the degree of liability exposure
3. Implementing corrective actions to minimize liability exposure in high-risk areas or activities[3]

Much of the work recommended in that program has been addressed in the preceding materials in this book, but the reader may wish to study the program recommended by Orlikoff and Vanagunas for further guidance on reducing the risk of liability.

What we wish to do now, however, is provide our own board risk management checklist as a means of summarizing the counsel and caution that have gone before. Some of the things listed in figure 7-1 require work by individual directors, but others are things that directors are entitled to require be done for them. In this sense, they constitute a small bill of rights for directors, aimed at providing freedom from personal liability.

Figure 7-1. Sample Risk Management Checklist for the Board to Minimize Personal Liability Exposure

☐ Require that each item preceded by an asterisk in this checklist is compiled into a binder and provided to each director, with annual updates as appropriate, and require that the following additional material be provided as well:
- Charter and bylaws
- State statute under which corporation is organized
- Medical staff bylaws
- Conflict policy
- Board policies on authority to make expenditures
- Board committee appointments
- Major event dates—board and committee meetings, retreats, conflict-of-interest disclosure filing, board evaluations, annual medical staff reappointment
- State regulations or standards regarding governance and medical staff
- Most recent Joint Commission standards on governance

☐*Adopt and implement a board conflict-of-interest policy and procedure that embodies or goes beyond state corporation law requirements and that provides for annual reporting through a disclosure questionnaire.

Continued on next page

Figure 7-1. Continued

- ☐ While serving as a director, don't do business with the corporation directly or indirectly through the sale of products or services to the corporation or the purchase of any of its assets.
- ☐*Require a periodic opinion from the hospital's lawyer regarding the conformance of the hospital organization's corporate documents with state corporation law.
- ☐ In major corporate transactions, seek legal review and written assurance that corporate action meets state law and corporate document requirements.
- ☐ Before authorizing asset transactions, be satisfied that they are in the best interests of the corporation and require a written opinion of counsel that the purpose for which the transaction is made is entirely legal and is within the authority of the board.
- ☐*Require that each director be advised in writing regarding state law provisions on director voting and the recording of director votes.
- ☐ Undertake an active board role in medical staff credentialing, using the board's activities in finance or other area of effective board performance as a model. Set initial goals:
  - ☐ Adopt a hospital medical staff credentialing mission or purpose statement describing what the board wants to accomplish with the hospital's medical staff credentialing system.
  - ☐ Instruct the hospital administrator to undertake a medical staff credentialing audit in order to obtain a baseline evaluation of the credentialing system and provide additional goals for board monitoring.
- ☐*Require that each director be provided with a description of state laws providing immunity for directors, a description of the corporation's bylaw provisions providing for director indemnification, and a description of the protection provided under the corporation's D&O insurance policy. Require an analysis pointing out specific gaps in the coverage of all of these protective devices and describing acts the board can take to close gaps or strengthen the protection.
- ☐*Require that each director be provided with a written explanation of how and when claims must be filed with the D&O insurance carrier when directors have notice of a liability claim against them.
- ☐ Take appropriate board action to maximize director protection under the state's immunity law or laws.
- ☐ Take appropriate board action to require director indemnification under the corporate bylaws.
- ☐ Take appropriate board action to expand the scope of D&O insurance protection and to ensure that full protection will continue to be provided after board membership has ended.
- ☐*Require that each director be provided with a list and analysis of director conduct that is prohibited by state law.
- ☐ Act with independence and record your vote.
- ☐ Require that the hospital administrator prepare an ongoing director education program underwritten by the corporation, provide adequate funds for its support, and require that all directors participate actively in the program as a condition of board membership.

Closing the Door on Liability

Under and subject to the law, a hospital's board of directors is its supreme authority. With few exceptions the law provides directors with the full power and authority necessary to carry out the duties it imposes on them. Hospital directors who exercise their rights and powers and who act with care, loyalty, and obedience to the laws and rules governing their conduct will have done just about everything possible to avoid, prevent, and protect against personal liability in board service.

What remains to be done in this book is to look at the five activities that are so critical to effective board performance that they are called the Five Commandments of Hospital Governance. Hospital boards that obey the commandments do more than build simple shelters to protect themselves from the liability wolf; they make their houses out of brick.

□ *References*

1. *Resolution of Conflicts of Interest in Health Care Institutions.* Chicago: American Hospital Association, 1975.
2. Illinois Revised Statutes, chapter 32, paragraph 108.65(b).
3. Orlikoff, J. E., and Vanagunas, A. M. *Malpractice Prevention and Liability Control for Hospitals.* Chicago: American Hospital Publishing, 1988, pp. 101–11.

Chapter 8

Five Commandments of Hospital Governance

Remember this, do that, careful here, caution there. Hospital directors are inundated—some would say plagued—with advice, information, and checklists, and your author feels some guilt by adding to the baggage. Is it possible for anyone to remember all these things? Unfortunately, try as we may, it is impossible to distill all that is important into a few, simple, memorable points of guidance that will suffice. The best we can do is to try to be comprehensive in our identification and to describe things in terms that are clear and comprehensible.

Still, in the author's experience, there are five areas of involvement that are fundamental for hospital boards of all kinds. If directors excel in these areas, they will do much to ensure effective board performance, probably the most important of all measures for avoiding director liability. These areas translate into the Five Commandments of Hospital Governance.

The First Commandment: Determine and Plan for Carrying Out the Mission of the Hospital

Laurence Peter put it best in *The Peter Principle:* "If you don't know where you're going, you will probably end up somewhere else." This sums up the purpose of the hospital corporation's mission statement: to serve as its North Star, its guiding light. Together with a strategic plan, a facilities master plan, and an annual business or operating plan, among others, the mission statement should provide the reference point for board decisions, especially the big ones. Good mission statements, which are followed and reflected in other planning documents, can help keep hospital managers and boards from doing goofy things, from flying off on wild tangents and harebrained schemes such as opening Pizza Power! pepperoni palaces.

As often as not, however, boards short themselves in this area. Mission statements are viewed as nice, but not essential. They tend toward soft words and warm feelings, for example: "The mission of Tiny General Hospital is to provide loving care in times of need." And they tend to be general in the extreme, for example: "The mission of Titanic Medical Center is to survive!" And even when they are good and really state what the organization is all about, they tend to be put away and forgotten.

More specific planning tools don't always fare much better. Despite the clear utility of strategic plans, facilities plans, and operating plans, boards have not always shown that they fully appreciate their importance. Indeed, history proves that when times were good and permitted business as usual, hospitals could get along fine without necessarily knowing where they were going. But times have changed dramatically.

Hospital board agendas today are crowded with items intended to improve viability, such as proposals for alliances and affiliations, new clinical programs, program discontinuance, facility modifications, and physician bonding programs. These are big items that can carry big price tags and alter the course of the hospital irretrievably. How are boards to judge, evaluate, and prioritize these and countless similar items on which the hospital's survival may someday hinge without the reference point of a clear mission backed up with thoughtful planning tools? Difficult to do, and because they are so difficult, they can result in serious mistakes that ultimately harm the corporation.

It is hard to imagine an experienced hospital director who hasn't participated in and witnessed these unguided actions and the resulting mistakes at one time or another. Land or facilities decisions are made before completion of a new or updated facilities plan. A few months or a few years later, it becomes evident that the land where the new parking tower is being built should really have been used for a medical office building or an outpatient surgical facility. Or the facilities plan fails to reflect program elements of the strategic plan.

Or the strategic plan is thrown to the wind when the board is asked to consider the start-up of a hot new program or the discontinuance of an old program that is central to the mission of the organization. Or a hospital affiliation is considered and approved without any look at how it corresponds with the mission or the strategic plan, and the medical staff, which helped build and has relied on the strategic plan to chart its own course, is outraged.

These things happen all the time in the hospital field. When they happen frequently at a single hospital, they increase the likelihood that a corporate disaster will occur. By putting a good mission and follow-up planning in place and sticking to the mission and the plans, boards reduce the likelihood of disaster by a considerable margin.

This is not a book on mission and planning, and no attempt will be made here to provide a detailed description of mission and planning development processes. Although they may seem obvious, however, a few things need to be said. A good mission statement describing *for what* the organization exists and *where it is headed* is essential. It should be general enough not to need frequent revision, but specific enough to provide guidance. And it should be comprehensible. Soft and fuzzy just doesn't make it when survival is at stake. Each director should be able to read the corporation's mission statement and say with confidence, "I've read it. I understand it. I know what we're here for, and I know where we want to go."

The mission statement should be on the table, not just when decisions are to be made, but whenever managers or directors get new notions in their noggins and start the process of developing proposals. When proposals finally are laid out for board consideration, part of the laying-out process should include the explanation of how they tie in to and support the mission.

The same process should be used in the development and revision of strategic, facilities, and operating plans, and, of course, these plans should play a central role in proposal development and consideration. Anything less leaves the board and the organization adrift.

The board's role in mission development and planning is not one of putting pen to paper. Most of that task belongs to administration. The board's job is one of setting goals, providing resources, reviewing and correcting the goals, and then, perhaps most important, making sure that the results are used by both management and governance. These are big jobs, and they require a good deal of board time on an ongoing basis. They call for a standing committee that can devote the time and develop the knowledge and expertise to do the job well.

The evaluation of the programs, projects, and other proposals of management against the standards of the corporation's mission and plans is an essential policy function of the board. Success in fulfilling the mission of the corporation depends largely on the availability of resources, a matter that may be beyond the board's control. But planning the use of the resources that are available is squarely within the board's power. This is one of the board's primary roles.

The Second Commandment: Provide for Qualified Management and Monitor Its Performance

The board defines the mission. Management is responsible for the mission's execution. As an old Chinese proverb says, "It is not enough to aim. You must hit." Finding and keeping a skilled chief executive officer (CEO) is solely the responsibility of the board. In large measure, the success of the board in responding to its duties will depend on its success in this endeavor.

The task doesn't end, however, with the payment of the recruiter's fee and the decorating of the executive's office. The directors must clearly define the role and performance goals of the CEO and grant the executive the full range of authority needed to carry them out.

Compensation of the CEO likewise falls within the board's purview. The board must educate itself regarding compensation arrangements and amounts for hospital management and take steps on a regular basis to ensure that its own CEO compensation package is competitive. And the board must monitor the performance of the CEO against objective and meaningful criteria covering all aspects of the executive's job.

Finally, the board must also discipline itself to prevent individual directors from engaging in petty backbiting and meddling in day-to-day operating matters. There is no surer way to drive out a skilled manager than to undercut or otherwise fail to support his or her authority.

The board's duty here is difficult and raises the dilemma mentioned much earlier in this book—that of entrusting executive management to managers while bearing ultimate responsibility for the affairs of the corporation. In a sense, the board must *know* the executive's job so that expectations as well as judgment of performance are realistic and meaningful.

Although the board can and should judge and counsel management, it should not substitute its efforts to make up for management's shortcomings. To do so is to misplace priorities. The only reasonable solution to continued poor performance by management is new management.

The Third Commandment: Ensure High Quality of Care

What doctors do and don't do has a greater impact on hospitals than almost anything else imaginable. Hospitals can be perfect in all other respects, but if high quality and efficiency are missing from the medical staff, the hospital will suffer the same fate. Thus, ensuring a high-quality medical staff is of such importance that it forces its way into the top priorities of the board. The board's tool for ensuring a high-quality medical staff is the hospital medical staff credentialing system.

Traditionally, this is the least understood and most poorly performed of all of the critical board functions. Boards have been led to believe that they are doing their job if they delegate the function to the medical staff. Nothing could be farther from the truth.

Although certain peer review activities relating to credentialing are appropriately delegated to the medical staff under various laws and standards, it is a grievous error to conclude that the board's role is merely accessory. Directors must educate themselves to understand the complex relationships between the medical staff and the hospital and the bases and processes of credentialing and quality assurance.

But this is not enough. Boards must also ensure that credentialing and quality assurance systems are provided with adequate personnel and resources. The board must establish a statement of purposes and goals for quality assurance and credentialing systems and monitor performance against them. As in the case of the hospital's financial systems, the board should provide for independent audits of the systems so that their strengths and weaknesses can be identified and corrective work can be undertaken. Ultimately, the board must do those things that give it a reasonable basis for confidence that the systems work in achieving their purposes.

Also important in today's competitive environment is the need for the board to play a role in building the medical staff and gaining its loyalty. It is not enough to attend the annual medical staff golf outing. The board must learn about and understand the pressures confronting doctors: professional liability, managed care, and other competitive medical delivery modes changing the health care marketplace. It must be involved in the planning and development of programs to assist doctors in responding to these pressures, for how the doctors respond will have a profound impact on the hospital itself.

This overall medical staff affairs function is so difficult, complex, and time-consuming that it merits the designation and the appointment of an active board standing committee, the members of which can gain the specialized knowledge necessary to deal in this arena and devote the time necessary to doing this critical job well.

The Fourth Commandment: Provide for the Financial Viability of the Hospital

Mark Twain was fond of pointing out that there are two times in life when people should not speculate: One is when they can't afford to; the other is when they can. In today's hospital world, the most dangerous form of speculation is a board's failure to manage the hospital's financial affairs. Fortunately, however, this is an area in which hospital boards frequently excel.

Hospital boards commonly seek out new directors who come to the board with ready-made expertise in treasury and financial management, and boards take steps to educate other directors whose knowledge may not be so broad. Maintaining this high level of specialized knowledge is absolutely necessary for good board performance.

Successful boards make sure that the hospital has first-rate financial managers, and they provide those managers with the resources they need to do their jobs. Successful boards also set realistic financial goals that tie in to the mission and plans of the organization. They review and act on capital and operating budgets in light of those goals, and they closely monitor ongoing financial performance in relation to the budget.

Boards that are strong in finance also oversee the development of financial control policies, set standards for and monitor investments, safeguard gifts and endowments, and play an active role in considering capital financing. Finally, these boards provide for an annual independent audit of the hospital corporation's financial systems and practices to ensure their validity and to point out needed changes.

Boards that do these things don't feel compelled to dig into and attempt to perform financial operations. They have a reasonable basis for being confident that the hospital's financial functions and systems are all that they should be. But failure to do these things can spell doom for the hospital corporation. The best board performance in finance may not save a hospital placed in jeopardy by market conditions, but lack of close attention can lead to financial failure. The duty of care dictates the role of the board in this area.

The Fifth Commandment: Understand Your Job and Equip Yourselves to Do It Well

There is no quick and easy way for hospital directors to learn what the job of the board—the job of governance—is all about. Certain aspects of the job become evident in short order: read minutes and reports; become familiar with jargon, relationships, and issues important to the hospital; vote on matters. But understanding the role of the board is an elusive task that brings to mind a poem by Tennyson:

> Flower in the crannied wall,
> I pluck you out of the crannies,
> I hold you here, root and all in my hand,
> Little flower — but *if* I could understand
> What you are, root and all, and all in all,
> I should know what God and man is.

There are, nonetheless, a number of steps that boards can take that will be useful in the quest for this understanding of the "all in all" and that will enable them to improve their effectiveness. These are selection, specialization, education, and evaluation. Thus, we end this book in a most appropriate way—by focusing on the all-important development of the hospital board of directors.

Selection of Board Members

Who makes the best director? The author has asked this question many times but has never received a consistent response. If there is any consensus at all, it is that broad knowledge of issues important to successful management of a hospital corporation is an essential characteristic for effective board performance. A board composed of responsible, experienced, and hardworking individuals with a wide and balanced spectrum of knowledge, backgrounds, and styles can provide invaluable advice, guidance, and counsel to management. Such a board stands a good chance of succeeding in the critical governance functions.

The process of selecting new directors is the starting point for ensuring continuance of an effective board. No board can expect that all new directors will know everything about everything, but careful selection can prevent the appointment of new directors who know nothing about anything, who are unwilling to make necessary commitments, or who are incapable of working constructively with other directors, managers, and the medical staff.

The process of selecting new directors is so important that it, too, merits a standing committee for the review and nomination of candidates. The committee and the board as a whole should develop director criteria beyond those found in the corporation's bylaws that are aimed at providing a balance of director skills and knowledge that will fortify the board and place it in a position to provide insights and assistance to management.

Specialization through Board Committees

Boards should make prudent use of board committees as a tool to foster specialized knowledge among directors and to spread the work of governance. The complexity of today's hospital organizations and health care environment renders it impossible for even the brightest, most dedicated, experienced, and resourceful director to master all issues coming before hospital boards.

The task can be accomplished only by dividing the work load among directors and allowing directors to develop areas of specialized expertise through participation in committees. Of particular importance are committees for planning, finance, medical staff affairs, and nominations. In larger organizations or organizations with special needs, committees for personnel, marketing, buildings and grounds, and others may also be appropriate.

Education of Board Members

Confucius once pointed out that learning without thought is labor lost but that thought without learning is perilous. Attempting to govern modern health care organizations in ignorance of the laws, principles, protocols, and issues affecting decisions, and without a sound basis for predicting outcomes, will invariably lead to poor decisions and bad results. Boards must implement policies and programs for education of the lay directors entrusted with the direction of the corporation, and diligent directors must set out to learn as much as they can about the subjects important to hospital governance.

All board members, for example, should gain a basic understanding of health care finance, and members of the finance committee should strive to excel in this area. Likewise, all directors should develop a general knowledge of the relationship between the medical staff and the hospital and of medical staff credentialing and quality assurance. Members of the board's medical staff affairs committee should acquire in-depth knowledge of these matters. Anecdotal knowledge of these and other subjects is often worse than no knowledge at all.

Orientation sessions and materials, retreats, seminars, regular guest speaker events, books, periodicals, and other continuing education devices must be sponsored and underwritten by the hospital corporation for the educational benefit of directors. Good board education is not cheap, but hospital spending to educate directors (who most frequently work for free) is typically only a fraction of amounts spent for the education of hospital employees (who are paid to know their jobs). Something is wrong in this equation. Without a concerted effort in this area, the education of the hospital's directors will always be inadequate, and only with luck will the board meet its legal duty of care.

Self-Evaluation and Remedial Action

How the board and the individual directors do in fulfilling their responsibilities can be judged only through a periodic and systematic process of self-evaluation and peer review. There are many tools available commercially to assist boards in undertaking self-assessment, and board evaluation is a requirement of the Joint Commission on Accreditation of Healthcare Organizations.

Submitting to the process, however, is not enough. The results of the process must be used to shore up performance. Weak directors can work harder to improve their contributions. Methods for improving board organization, communications, meeting formats, and educational opportunities can be developed and implemented.

Done with skill and treated as a priority, the self-evaluation task can result in improved board efficiency, productivity, and effectiveness. Done poorly, it can be an exercise in tedium. But directors who shy away from the mirror of self-evaluation and prefer to look only at their feet, run the risk of eventually seeing them covered with mud.

Conclusion

Mission, management selection, medical staff quality, finance, and board development. These are the themes covered by the Five Commandments of Hospital Governance. They are the essence of the board's job.

When hospital directors carry out these commandments and serve their corporations with loyalty, care, and obedience, they do their jobs well. When, in addition, they cloak themselves with the full power of the "three eyes" and focus special attention on the issues that are known to carry risk, they are doing everything possible to prevent troubles with director liability from ever entering their boardrooms.

Appendix A

Standards for Hospital Governing Bodies from the Joint Commission on Accreditation of Healthcare Organizations

Standard

GB.1 An organized governing body, or designated persons so functioning, is responsible for establishing policy, maintaining quality patient care, and providing for institutional management and planning.*

Required Characteristics

GB.1.1 The governing body adopts bylaws in accordance with its legal accountability and its responsibility to the patient population served.*

GB.1.2 The bylaws specify at least the following:*

GB.1.2.1 The role and purpose of the hospital.

GB.1.2.2 The duties and responsibilities of the governing body.*

GB.1.2.3 The process for selecting members of the governing body.

Reprinted with permission from the 1991 *Accreditation Manual for Hospitals,* copyright 1990 by the Joint Commission on Accreditation of Healthcare Organizations, Oakbrook Terrace, IL, pp. 49–53.

*The asterisked items are key factors in the accreditation decision process. For an explanation of the use of the key factors, see "Using the Manual," page ix, of the *Accreditation Manual for Hospitals,* 1991 edition.

Note: "Governing Body" is defined as: "The individual(s), group or agency that has ultimate authority and responsibility for overall operation of the organization."

GB.1.2.3.1 The bylaws specify criteria for the selection of members of the governing body.*

GB.1.2.4 The governing body's organizational structure, including at least
GB.1.2.4.1 the mechanism for selecting officers;

GB.1.2.4.2 the responsibilities of officers;

GB.1.2.4.3 the procedures for meetings;

GB.1.2.4.4 the composition and responsibilities of governing body committees, if any;* and

GB.1.2.4.5 the inclusion of medical staff members on governing body committees that deliberate issues affecting the discharge of medical staff responsibilities.*

GB.1.2.5 The relationship of responsibilities of the governing body and
GB.1.2.5.1 any authority superior to the governing body, if such exists;*

GB.1.2.5.2 the chief executive officer;* and

GB.1.2.5.3 the medical staff.*

GB.1.2.6 The requirement for the establishment of a medical staff.*

GB.1.2.7 The requirement for the establishment of auxiliary organizations, if applicable.

GB.1.2.8 The mechanism for adopting the governing body bylaws.

GB.1.2.9 The mechanism for review and revision of the bylaws.

GB.1.3 When not legally prohibited, members of the medical staff are eligible for full membership on the governing body in the same manner as other individuals.

GB.1.4 The medical staff has the right of representation (through attendance and voice), by one or more medical staff members selected by the medical staff, at meetings of the governing body.*

GB.1.5 There is a systematic and effective mechanism for communication between members of the governing body, the administration, and the medical staff.*

    GB.1.5.1 In addition, there is a systematic and effective mechanism for communication between the hospital's governing body, administration, and medical staff and the governing bodies and management of any health care delivery organizations that are corporately and functionally related to the hospital.*

GB.1.6 Any auxiliary organizations and individual volunteers delineate their purpose and function for approval by the governing body.

    GB.1.6.1 The governing body approves the bylaws that delineate the purpose and function of any auxiliary organizations.

    GB.1.6.2 The governing body establishes a mechanism for services provided by individual volunteers.

GB.1.7 A record of governing body proceedings is maintained.*

GB.1.8 The governing body provides for institutional planning.

    GB.1.8.1 The administration, the medical staff, the nursing department/service, other departments/services, and appropriate advisers participate in the planning process.

GB.1.9 The governing body approves an annual operating budget, develops a long-term capital expenditure plan as required by applicable law and regulation, and monitors implementation of the plan.*

GB.1.10 The governing body appoints a chief executive officer.*

    GB.1.10.1 The chief executive officer is qualified for his responsibilities through education and experience.*

        GB.1.10.1.1 The governing body designates a mechanism for monitoring the chief executive officer's performance.*

GB.1.11 The medical staff executive committee makes recommendations directly to the governing body for its approval.*

    GB.1.11.1 Such recommendations pertain to at least the following:

        GB.1.11.1.1 The structure of the medical staff;

GB.1.11.1.2 The mechanism used to review credentials and to delineate individual clinical privileges;

GB.1.11.1.3 Individual medical staff membership;

GB.1.11.1.4 Specific clinical privileges for each eligible individual;

GB.1.11.1.5 The organization of the quality assurance activities of the medical staff as well as the mechanism used to conduct, evaluate, and revise such activities;

GB.1.11.1.6 The mechanism by which membership on the medical staff may be terminated; and

GB.1.11.1.7 The mechanism for fair-hearing procedures.

GB.1.12 Any differences in recommendations concerning medical staff appointments, reappointments, terminations of appointments, and the granting or revision of clinical privileges are resolved within a reasonable period of time by the governing body and the medical staff.*

GB.1.13 The governing body acts on recommendations concerning medical staff appointments, reappointments, terminations of appointments, and the granting or revision of clinical privileges within a reasonable period of time, as specified in the bylaws of the medical staff.*

GB.1.14 The governing body requires that only a member of the medical staff with admitting privileges may admit a patient to the hospital and that such individuals may practice only within the scope of the privileges granted by the governing body, and that each patient's general medical condition is the responsibility of a qualified physician member of the medical staff.*

GB.1.15 The governing body requires a process or processes designed to assure that all individuals who provide patient care services, but who are not subject to the medical staff privilege delineation process, are competent to provide such services.*

GB.1.15.1 The quality of patient care services provided by these individuals is reviewed as part of the hospital's quality assurance program.*

Appendix A

GB.1.16 The governing body requires a process or processes designed to assure that all individuals responsible for the assessment, treatment, or care of patients are competent in the following, as appropriate to the ages of the patients served:*

GB.1.16.1 the ability to obtain information and interpret information in terms of the patient's needs;

GB.1.16.2 a knowledge of growth and development; and

GB.1.16.3 an understanding of the range of treatment needed by these patients.

GB.1.17 The governing body requires mechanisms to assure the provision of one level of patient care in the hospital.*

GB.1.17.1 The governing body requires mechanisms to assure that all patients with the same health problem are receiving the same level of care in the hospital.*

GB.1.18 The governing body requires the medical staff and staffs of the departments/services to implement and report on the activities and mechanisms for monitoring and evaluating the quality of patient care, for identifying and resolving problems, and for identifying opportunities to improve patient care.*

GB.1.18.1 The governing body, through the chief executive officer, supports these activities and mechanisms.*

GB.1.19 The governing body provides for resources and support systems for the quality assurance functions and risk management functions related to patient care and safety.*

GB.1.20 The governing body holds the medical staff responsible for the development, adoption, and periodic review of medical staff bylaws and rules and regulations that are consistent with hospital policy and with any applicable legal or other requirements.*

GB.1.20.1 The medical staff bylaws and rules and regulations that have been adopted by the medical staff are subject to, and effective upon, approval by the governing body; approval is not unreasonably withheld.*

GB.1.21 The governing body evaluates its own performance.

GB.1.22 The governing body's bylaws and/or rules and regulations specify the authority and responsibility of each level of the organization in respect to*

GB.1.22.1 quality of care;

GB.1.22.2 quality assurance mechanisms;

GB.1.22.3 credentials review and privilege delineation;

GB.1.22.4 selection of the hospital's governing body;

GB.1.22.5 selection of the hospital's chief executive officer and other key management staff;

GB.1.22.6 selection of medical staff department chairmen;

GB.1.22.7 planning of hospital services;

GB.1.22.8 development and approval of the hospital's budget; and

GB.1.22.9 review of the governing body's performance.

Standard

GB.2 The governing body avoids conflict of interest.*

Required Characteristics

GB.2.1 The governing body provides for full disclosure of the ownership and control of the hospital and of any health care delivery organizations that are corporately and functionally related to the hospital.*

GB.2.2 The governing body develops and implements a written conflict-of-interest policy that includes guidelines for the resolution of any existing or apparent conflict of interest.

Standard

GB.3 All members of the governing body understand and fulfill their responsibilities.*

Required Characteristics

GB.3.1 All new members of the governing body participate in an orientation program.

GB.3.2 All members of the governing body are provided information relating to the governing body's responsibility for quality care and the hospital's quality assurance program.

GB.3.3 A program of continuing education is available to all members of the governing body.

Appendix B

State Statutes That Provide Immunity (Either Directly or Indirectly) for Directors or Trustees of Hospital Boards

1. *Alabama:* Ala. Code §10-11-1 (1987) provides immunity for uncompensated officers, directors, or trustees of nonprofit corporations provided that their conduct is not willful, wanton, grossly negligent, or fraudulent.

2. *Arkansas:* Ark. Stat. Ann. §16-120-102 (1989 Supp.) provides immunity for officers, directors, or trustees of nonprofit corporations or governmental entities from tort liability. §16-120-103 lists the exemptions: ordinary or gross negligence and intentional torts.

3. *California:* Cal. Corporations Code §9247 (1990) provides immunity from personal liability for volunteer (uncompensated) directors or officers for negligence. The statute exempts recklessness, wanton, intentional, or grossly negligent conduct, self-dealing, and actions brought by the attorney general. In addition, the nonprofit organization must have liability insurance for directors and officers, or the individual must have a policy.

    Cal. Public Health Code §24001.5 (1990 Supp.) provides immunity for officers, directors, or trustees of nonprofit medical centers who serve without compensation. The statute exempts self-dealing, conflicts of interest, actions brought by a beneficiary of a trust, and willful, wanton acts. Furthermore, the hospital must have liability insurance and it must be in force at the time of the negligent act or omission.

4. *Colorado:* Colo. Rev. Stat. §13-21-116 (1987) provides immunity for noncompensated directors or officers. The statute exempts wanton and willful acts.

5. *Delaware:* Del. Code Ann. tit. 10, §8133 (1988 Supp.) provides immunity for volunteer trustees, officers, or directors of nonprofit corporations.

The statute exempts negligence while operating a motor vehicle and willful, wanton, or grossly negligent conduct.

6. *Florida:* Fla. Stat. §617.0285 (1990 Supp.) provides immunity for directors, officers, and trustees of nonprofit corporations. The statute exempts violations of the criminal law, unlawful conduct, self-dealing, recklessness, or any act committed in bad faith or with a malicious, willful, or wanton disregard.

7. *Georgia:* Ga. Code Ann. §105-114 provides that a person serving with or without compensation as a member, officer, director, or trustee of any board of a nonprofit institution is immune unless he or she was acting with willful or wanton misconduct.

8. *Hawaii:* Haw. Rev. Stat. §4158-158.5 (1989 Supp.) provides immunity for directors, officers, or trustees of nonprofit corporations who are uncompensated. The statute exempts gross negligence.

9. *Idaho:* Idaho Code §6-1605 (1990) provides immunity for officers, directors, and volunteers of nonprofit corporations and organizations who serve without compensation. The act exempts willful, wanton conduct, fraud, knowing violations of the law, intentional breaches of fiduciary duty, self-dealing, and any damages that arise from operation of a motor vehicle.

10. *Illinois:* Ill. Rev. Stat. ch. 32, §108.70 (1990) provides immunity for directors, officers, and persons who serve without compensation in nonprofit corporations or organizations. The statute exempts willful and wanton conduct.

11. *Indiana:* Ind. Code §34-4-11.5-2 (1990 Supp.) provides immunity for directors of government agencies, nonprofits, or corporations providing hospital services, emergency services, or medical research if they serve without compensation.

12. *Iowa:* Iowa Code §504A.101 (1990 Supp.) provides immunity for directors, officers, or volunteers of a nonprofit corporation as long as their acts do not involve breach of the duty of loyalty to the corporation, acts not in good faith, intentional misconduct, knowing violation of the law, or a transaction from which the individual derives personal benefit.

13. *Kansas:* Kan. Stat. Ann. §65-442 (1985) provides that there will be no liability for any member of the governing board or of a committee of the medical staff of a licensed medical care facility for any act, statement, or proceeding taken and performed within the scope of the duties unless he or she acted with malice.

§60-3601 provides immunity for volunteers of nonprofit organizations. Exempted from the statute are willful, wanton acts or intentional tortious conduct.

Appendix B

14. *Kentucky:* Ky. Rev. Stat. §411.200 (1990 Supp.) provides immunity for directors, officers, or trustees of nonprofit organizations who are not compensated. Exempted is willful or wanton misconduct.
15. *Louisiana:* La. Rev. Stat. Ann. §9-2792.1 (West 1990 Supp.) provides immunity for officers, trustees, or directors of nonprofit organizations who are not compensated. Exempted is willful or wanton misconduct.
    §9.2792 (1990 Supp.) provides immunity for a director or trustee of a nonprofit hospital.
16. *Maine:* Me. Rev. Stat. Ann. tit. 14, §158A (1990) provides immunity for directors, officers, or volunteers of nonprofit organizations who are not compensated.
17. *Maryland:* Md. Code Ann. §5-309.3 (1990) provides that licensed physicians and volunteers (officer, trustee, or other person who performs services without compensation) are not liable. The statute exempts willful and wanton conduct, gross negligence, and intentionally tortious conduct.
18. *Massachusetts:* Mass. Gen. L. §231:85W (1990) provides that officers and directors of charitable corporations (not-for-profit) who are not compensated are granted immunity. This immunity does not apply to intentional acts, grossly negligent acts, acts of omission committed in the course of commercial activity, or negligence in operating a motor vehicle.
19. *Michigan:* Mich. Comp. Laws Ann. §450.2209 (West 1990) provides that the articles of incorporation of a nonprofit corporation can enable immunization of the volunteer director. The statute exempts intentional misconduct, knowing violation of the law, grossly negligent acts or omissions, and acts or omissions before January 1, 1988.
20. *Minnesota:* Minn. Stat. §317A:257 (1990 Supp.) provides immunity for directors, officers, and trustees of nonprofit organizations who serve without compensation. The statute exempts willful and wanton acts, breach of fiduciary duty, causes of action based on federal law or express contractual obligations, breach of public pension plans, physical injury, and wrongful death.
21. *Mississippi:* Miss. Code Ann. §41-13-11 (1990 Supp.) provides immunity for members of the board of trustees, officers, agents, or employees of a community hospital if the hospital has liability insurance. Note this statute is not effective after October 1991.
22. *Missouri:* Mo. Rev. Stat. §537.117 (1988) provides that any officer or member of a governing body of a nonprofit corporation who is not compensated is immune. The immunity does not extend to intentional conduct, willful or wanton acts, or gross negligence.

23. *Montana:* Mont. Code Ann. §27-1-732 (1989) provides immunity for an officer, director, or volunteer of a nonprofit corporation. The statute exempts willful and wanton conduct.

24. *Nebraska:* Neb. Rev. Stat. §25-21.191 (1989) provides immunity for a director, officer, or trustee of a nonprofit corporation who is not compensated. The statute exempts willful and wanton conduct, conduct while operating a motor vehicle, and conduct impaired by alcohol or controlled substances.

25. *Nevada:* Nev. Rev. Stat. §41-480 (1986) provides immunity to an officer, trustee, or director of a nonprofit corporation. The statute exempts intentional misconduct, fraud, and knowing violations of the law.

26. *New Hampshire:* N.H. Rev. Stat. Ann. §508:16 (1989 Supp.) provides immunity for directors and officers who serve without compensation in nonprofit corporations. The statute exempts willful or wanton misconduct.

27. *New Jersey:* N.J. Rev. Stat. §2A:53A-7.1 (1987) provides immunity for persons serving nonprofit corporations and societies or associations organized for religious, charitable, educational, or hospital purposes, provided that they are uncompensated. The statute exempts willful, wanton, or grossly negligent acts, negligent operation of a motor vehicle, or reckless disregard of the duties imposed by the position.

28. *New Mexico:* N.M. Stat. Ann. §53-8-25.3 (1989 Supp.) provides immunity for members of the board of directors of a nonprofit corporation. The statute exempts breach or failure to perform duties, and the breach must constitute willful misconduct or recklessness. Immunity is limited to actions taken as a director at meetings of the board or a committee or by action of the directors at the meeting.

29. *New York:* N.Y. Not-for-Profit Corporation Law §720a (McKinney 1990 Supp.) provides immunity for directors, officers, or trustees of a nonprofit corporation who are not compensated. The statute excludes intentional acts or actions brought by the attorney general.

30. *North Carolina:* N.C. Gen. Stat. §131E-47.1 (1988) provides immunity for uncompensated directors, trustees or officers of a public hospital (defined as a hospital owned and operated by the state or a nonprofit). The statute exempts gross negligence, willful and wanton conduct, improper personal financial benefit, and operation of a motor vehicle.

31. *North Dakota:* N.D. Cent. Code §32-03-44 (1989 Supp.) provides immunity for directors, officers, or trustees of nonprofit corporations if they are acting in good faith with no willful misconduct or gross negligence. Furthermore, they may not be reimbursed in excess of $2,000 per year and may not be compensated.

Appendix B

32. *Ohio:* Ohio Rev. Code Ann. §2305.38 (1990) provides immunity for uncompensated officers, directors, and trustees of nonprofit corporations. The statute exempts willful, wanton, and tortious acts.

33. *Oklahoma:* Okla. Stat. tit. 32, §2612 (West 1990) provides immunity for directors, officers, or employees of nonprofit hospitals holding certificates of authority. Tit. 18, §866 provides immunity for directors of nonprofit corporations who are not compensated. The immunity does not extend to intentional torts or grossly negligent acts or omissions.

34. *Oregon:* Or. Rev. Stat. §65.369 (1989) provides immunity for directors, officers, and trustees of nonprofit organizations, including medical organizations or hospitals serving at a reduced cost. The statute exempts gross negligence and intentional acts.

35. *Pennsylvania:* Pa. Stat. Ann. tit. 42, §8364 (Purdon 1990 Supp.) provides immunity for directors of either for-profit or not-for-profit corporations by a vote of the majority of the shareholders. The statute exempts breaches of fiduciary duty that constitute self-dealing, willful misconduct or recklessness, criminal liability, and tax liability.

36. *Rhode Island:* R.I. Gen. Laws §7-6-9 (1989 Supp.) provides immunity for uncompensated directors or officers of nonprofit corporations. The statute exempts malicious, willful, and wanton misconduct.

37. *South Carolina:* S.C. Code Ann. §33-55-210 (1990) provides that any individual sustaining injury or dying because of a tortious act of an employee of a charitable organization can only recover against the charitable organization.

38. *South Dakota:* S.D. Codified Laws Ann. §47-23.29 (1990 Supp.) provides that noncompensated volunteers of nonprofit organizations, corporations, or hospitals or a government entity are immune. The statute exempts willful and wanton misconduct, and negligent operation of a motor vehicle (§47-23-30).

39. *Tennessee:* Tenn. Code Ann. §48-58-601 (1990 Supp.) provides directors, trustees, and members of governing bodies of nonprofit corporations, whether compensated or not, with immunity unless the individual's conduct is willful, wanton, or grossly negligent.

40. *Texas:* Tex. Civil Practice and Remedies Code Ann. §84.001-84.008 (Vernon 1990 Supp.) provides immunity for uncompensated directors, officers, or trustees of charitable organizations defined as nonprofits, including hospitals. The statute does not apply to intentional, willful, wanton, or reckless acts or operation of a motor vehicle.

41. *Utah:* Utah Code Ann. §63-30-3 (1989) provides government immunity for state-owned and operated health care facilities, but not for the employees thereof.

42. *Vermont:* Vt. Stat. Ann. tit. 12, §5781 (1989 Supp.) provides immunity for directors, officers, or trustees of nonprofit corporations who serve without compensation. The statute exempts gross negligence, intentional torts, and negligence in the operation of motor vehicles.

43. *Washington:* Wash. Rev. Code §24.03.025 (1990 Supp.) provides that the articles of incorporation of a nonprofit corporation can limit or eliminate the personal liability of a director of the corporation. Liability for acts or omissions involving intentional misconduct or knowing violation of the law or for any transaction in which the director receives personal benefit cannot be limited.

44. *West Virginia:* W.Va. Code §55-7C-3 (1990 Supp.) provides immunity for qualified directors (uncompensated directors who serve nonprofit organizations, including organizations that supply medical or hospital care). The statute exempts gross negligence and negligence in the operation of a motor vehicle.

45. *Wisconsin:* Wis. Stat. §181.287 (1989 Supp.) provides immunity for directors and officers of nonstock corporations. Exempted from the statute are willful failures to deal fairly with the corporation, violations of the criminal law, self-dealing, willful misconduct, civil or criminal proceedings brought by the government, and violations of state or federal law.

46. *Wyoming:* Wyo. Stat. §1-23-107 (1988 Supp.) provides immunity for members of the board of a nonprofit corporation. The statute exempts intentional torts and illegal acts.

Appendix C

State Statutes That Provide Immunity for Members of Peer Review Committees

1. *Alabama:* Ala. Code §34-24-361 (1990 Supp.)
2. *Alaska:* Alaska Stat. §18-23-020 (1986)
3. *Arizona:* Ariz. Rev. Stat. §36-445.02 (1989 Supp.)
4. *Arkansas:* Ark. Stat. Ann. §20-9-502 (1987)
5. *California:* Cal. Civil Code §43.7 (1990 Supp.)
6. *Colorado:* Colo. Rev. Stat. §12-36-118 (1990 Supp.)
7. *Delaware:* Del. Code Ann. §24-1768 (1988 Supp.)
8. *District of Columbia:* D.C. Code Ann. §32-503 (1981)
9. *Florida:* Fla. Stat. §766.101 (1990 Supp.)
10. *Georgia:* Ga. Code Ann. §84-7603 (1989 Supp.)
11. *Hawaii:* Haw. Rev. Stat. §671D.10 (1989 Supp.)
12. *Idaho:* Idaho Code §39-1392e (1985)
13. *Illinois:* Ill. Rev. Stat. ch. 111, §4400-5 (1989 Supp.)
14. *Indiana:* Ind. Code §34-4-12.6-3 (1983)
15. *Iowa:* Iowa Code §147.135 (1989)
16. *Kansas:* Kan. Stat. Ann. §65-4915 (1989 Supp.)
17. *Kentucky:* Ky. Rev. Stat. tit. 26, §311.377 (1988)
18. *Louisiana:* La. Rev. Stat. Ann. §13:3715.3 (1990 Supp.)

19. *Maine:* Me. Rev. Stat. Ann. tit. 24, §2511 (1990)
20. *Maryland:* Md. Code Ann. §14-603, 14-511 (1990 Supp.)
21. *Massachusetts:* Mass. Gen. L. tit. 111, §203, 204 (1990 Supp.)
22. *Michigan:* Mich. Comp. Laws Ann. §333.16244 (1990 Supp.)
23. *Minnesota:* Minn. Stat. §147.121 (1989)
24. *Mississippi:* Miss. Code Ann. §73-25-91 (1989)
25. *Missouri:* Mo. Rev. Stat. §537.035 (1988)
26. *Montana:* Mont. Code Ann. §37-2-201 (1989)
27. *Nebraska:* Neb. Rev. Stat. §25.12.121 (1989)
28. *Nevada:* Nev. Rev. Stat. §49.265 (1989 Supp.)
29. *New Hampshire:* N.H. Rev. Stat. Ann. §507:8-c (1983)
30. *New Jersey:* N.J. Rev. Stat. §24A:84A-22.10 (1987)
31. *New Mexico:* N.M. Stat. Ann. §61-6-16 (1989 Supp.)
32. *New York:* N.Y. Pub HE Law §2801-b (McKinney 1990 Supp.)
33. *North Carolina:* N.C. Gen. Stat. §90-21.22 (1989 Supp.)
34. *North Dakota:* N.D. Cent. Code §31-08-01 (1978)
35. *Ohio:* Ohio Rev. Code Ann. §2305.25 (Anderson 1989 Supp.)
36. *Oklahoma:* Okla. Stat. tit. 76, §24-29 (1990 Supp.)
37. *Pennsylvania:* Pa. Stat. Ann. tit. 63, §425.1 (1990 Supp.)
38. *Rhode Island:* R.I. Gen. Laws §5-37.3-7 (1989)
39. *South Carolina:* S.C. Code Ann. §40-71-10 (1989 Supp.)
40. *South Dakota:* S.D. Codified Laws Ann. §36-4-24 (1986)
41. *Tennessee:* Tenn. Code Ann. §63-6-219 (1990)
42. *Texas:* Tex. Civil Statutes §4495b (1990 Supp.)
43. *Utah:* Utah Code Ann. §58-12-25 (1990)
44. *Vermont:* Vt. Stat. Ann. tit. 26, §1442 (1989)
45. *Washington:* Wash. Rev. Code §4.24.240 (1988)
46. *West Virginia:* W.Va. Code §30-3-14 (1990 Supp.)
47. *Wisconsin:* Wis. Stat. ch. 146, §146.37 (1988)
48. *Wyoming:* Wyo. Stat. §35-17-103 (1988)